The Parents' Emergency Medical Guide

The Parents' Emergency Medical Guide

Robert Kaplan, M.D.

McGraw-Hill Book Company

New York St. Louis San Francisco Hamburg Mexico Toronto

Trademarks   Below is a list of trademarks used in this book, together with the firms in whose names the trademarks have been registered.

Slophyllin: William H. Rorer, Inc.
Quibron, Lytren, Prosobee: Mead Johnson & Co.
Theodur: Key Pharmaceuticals, Inc.
Benadryl, Agoral: Parke-Davis
Atarax: Roerig
Neo-Synephrine: Winthrop Consumer Products
Kondremul: Fisons Corp.
Pedialyte, Isomil: Ross Laboratories
Dove: Lever Brothers, Co.
Neutrogena: Neutrogena Corp.
Basis, Eucerin: Beiersdorf, Inc.
Lowila, Alpha-Keri: Westwood Pharmaceuticals, Inc.
Aveeno: Cooper Care, Inc.
Duofilm: Stiefel Laboratories, Inc.
Dramamine: Searle Consumer Products
Kaopectate: Upjohn

3 4 5 6 7 8 9 SEM SEM 8 7 6

ISBN 0-07-033536-2{PBK.}
ISBN 0-07-033556-7{H.C.}

Library of Congress Cataloging-in-Publication Data

Kaplan, Robert E.
  The parents' emergency medical guide.

  1. Pediatric emergencies.   2. Children—Diseases—
Popular works.   I. Title.   [DNLM: 1. Emergencies—in
infancy & childhood—popular works.   2. Emergency
Medicine—in infancy & childhood—popular works.
WS 200 K17p]
RJ370.K36 1987   618.92'0025   86-10339
ISBN 0-07-033536-2(PBK)
ISBN 0-07-033556-7(HC)

Illustrations by Laura Hartman
Editing Supervisor: Margery Luhrs
Book design by M.R.P. Design

To Jean

Contents

Contents

Contents

Contents

Acknowledgments

There are many individuals who have assisted in the creation of this book. My family has been a constant source of support and encouragement. The project would never have taken off without the invaluable assistance of Abbey, Gloria, and Sheldon Zalaznick.

Jackie Conroy and Dr. Alan Kornberg were extremely helpful in reviewing the entire manuscript. Others who reviewed sections of the book and provided expert advice include: Dr. Norman Ellerstein, Dr. Leo Heitlinger, Dr. Dennis Nadler, Dr. Thomas Rossi, Dr. Saul Kaplan, Dr. Aaron Kaplan, Amy Doerr, and Dr. Robert Welliver.

I would also like to thank Philippa Brophy and Tom Miller for their tremendous help and support.

I will always carry the memory of my late mother's love and warmth for children, and her great insight and marvel regarding growth and development. It is because of her that I became a pediatrician. My father lovingly and rigorously taught me how to write, and gave me the impetus to be an author.

My daughters, Anna and Leah, have taught me more

about children and pediatrics than four years of medical school, and several years of training.

It is because of my wife, Jean, that we have a very special family. Jean is a wonderful mother, and I have learned a great deal by her example. She has aided me throughout this project with her insights, comments, and most importantly her tolerance and understanding during the many hours I was locked in the "computer room."

Introduction

Parents know that raising children is a wonderful yet sometimes difficult experience. Children get sick, and they get hurt. These situations can be complicated and confusing. When faced with a specific emergency, we all find clear and practical advice helpful. Aunts, uncles, grandparents, great-grandparents, cousins, friends, neighbors, teachers, and baby-sitters all take part in raising children. This book is written not only for parents but for anyone who takes care of children.

I began to think about writing this book shortly after Anna, our first child, was born. I was in the midst of changing her diaper one night, and she was crying pretty hard. It took her a little longer than usual to settle down. This concerned me. In fact, I became scared. I began going through a mental checklist of all the possible things that could be bothering her. Was she wet? Was she hungry? Was she too hot? Was she too cold? Was she overtired? Was she sick? As it turned out, she was just wet. However, I realized that even when one has the benefit of highly specialized medical training, caring for children can at times be an awesome task.

This book gives a practical approach to common problems and emergencies which involve children. This is not an encyclopedia or textbook. It is a manual designed to help you make the proper decisions when faced with a real emergency.

In writing this book, I identified the options that are available and the decisions that must be made when one is managing specific medical problems commonly encountered with infants and children. I then organized the different scenarios in a step-by-step fashion and constructed a "map" for each individual problem. Each map helps you make rapid decisions in a specific situation and directs you in terms of taking specific first-aid or other measures and seeking medical attention. There is a sample map on page xxvi.

Parents often agonize at three o'clock in the morning over whether they should call the doctor immediately or wait for several hours until someone will be in the office. There is nothing more embarrassing for parents than being put down as "overanxious" by a physician or a nurse. More important, you want to avoid being labeled as parents who "cry wolf" at the most minor problem, because you want to be believed when you have a real problem on your hands.

If you are concerned about your child's welfare and it is one o'clock on a Sunday morning, you need to know confidently that you are handling the situation properly. The maps will help you in this regard. They will let you know *if* you need to call immediately, *when* to call later, and *whom* to call when medical assistance is necessary. Your options will usually include the following:

- Observing your child for a certain period of time.
- Calling your doctor or clinic during regular office or phone hours. "Phone hours" are those times set aside by your doctor or clinic to answer your questions over the telephone.
- Calling your doctor or clinic or an emergency room immediately.
- Going directly to an emergency room.

- Calling 911 (or Operator) for an ambulance. In most areas of the United States, 911 is the designated "emergency telephone number," and if you live in one of these areas, you should use it. However, there are some areas (mostly rural ones), where 911 is still not in use; if you live in one of these areas, you should call Operator (the zero on your telephone, often marked "OPER") during an emergency.

You will notice that the book is divided into four parts: Part I, "Emergencies," Part II, "Common Problems and Concerns," Part III, "Prevention," and Part IV, "Medical Terms." It is best to read carefully about emergencies (in Part I) and prevention (in Part III) now. Reading about possible emergencies will make things easier for you when you find yourself in an actual one, and following the instructions given in Part III will help you prevent most emergencies by making your home as safe as possible for your child. You can read about specific problems and areas of concern in Part II as they come up, and you can look up medical terms and definitions in Part IV as needed.

A WORD ABOUT *He* AND *She*

Throughout the book I have alternated the use of *he* and *she*. For example, "she has a cough," "he has a diaper rash." I have abandoned, like so many other authors, the arbitrary convention of using *he* exclusively. This convention of male exclusivity has lost its validity. I was quite tempted, as the father of two wonderful girls, to refer solely to *she*; however, that would not have been fair either.

How to Use a Map in This Book

What follows is an explanation of how a map in this book works.

Your 8-year-old son has hurt himself playing basketball. He comes running into the house, crying, holding his right hand. He tells you that he "jammed" his finger. You look at his hand and notice that he has injured his right middle finger.

The map on the next page outlines what might happen and the decisions you can make.

You start with the top box and work your way down the page following the arrows. When you come to a box that has two exit arrows, you have to follow the "yes" path or the "no" path. In this example, if the injured finger was bent, crooked, discolored, or very swollen, you would follow the "yes" path and call your doctor or clinic immediately or take your child to an emergency room. If the finger was not bent, crooked, discolored, or very swollen, you would follow the "no" path and continue down the map. Your final plan of action in this example would depend on whether your child could make a fist with the injured hand.

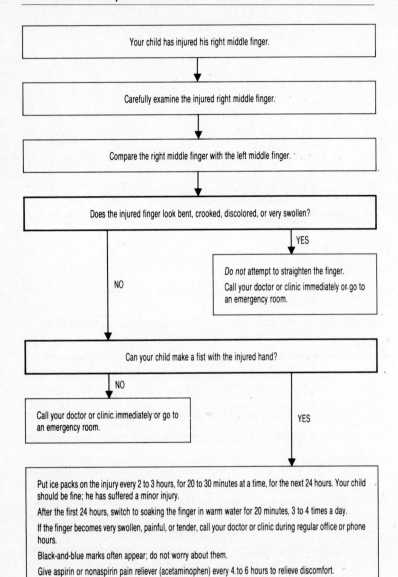

Your child has injured his right middle finger.

Carefully examine the injured right middle finger.

Compare the right middle finger with the left middle finger.

Does the injured finger look bent, crooked, discolored, or very swollen?

YES

Do not attempt to straighten the finger.

Call your doctor or clinic immediately or go to an emergency room.

NO

Can your child make a fist with the injured hand?

NO

Call your doctor or clinic immediately or go to an emergency room.

YES

Put ice packs on the injury every 2 to 3 hours, for 20 to 30 minutes at a time, for the next 24 hours. Your child should be fine; he has suffered a minor injury.

After the first 24 hours, switch to soaking the finger in warm water for 20 minutes, 3 to 4 times a day.

If the finger becomes very swollen, painful, or tender, call your doctor or clinic during regular office or phone hours.

Black-and-blue marks often appear; do not worry about them.

Give aspirin or nonaspirin pain reliever (acetaminophen) every 4 to 6 hours to relieve discomfort.

Have your child rest the injured area for at least 2 days, and then begin to reuse the finger gradually.

I. *Emergencies*

How to Handle Emergencies

For parents, almost nothing creates a greater sense of fear and helplessness than the experience of being confronted suddenly with a seriously ill or injured child.

It's impossible to plan for all emergencies, but you can take precautionary measures before emergencies happen. Reading through the specific MAPS in Part I now will help you deal with an emergency should it happen. Listed below are several tips for handling emergencies.

1. Start by Trying to Prevent Them

I repeat this theme over and over because it is so important. Most childhood injuries are preventable, and most occur either in cars or at home; Part III, "Prevention," discusses the steps to take in much greater detail. However, here are some general guidelines to get you started:

- Make your car and home safe for an infant or child. Do this by always using car safety seats and safety belts, and by "child-proofing" your home.
- Always arrange for infants and children to be properly supervised.
- *Learn CPR* (cardiopulmonary resuscitation). Most often used in adult emergencies, this technique can save a child's life also.

2. Don't Panic

This sounds simple and obvious, but it is crucial. Try and take things step by step. This will help you keep things under control.

One thing that often frightens people is the sight of blood. Remember, it only takes a small amount of blood to cause a very large and frightening stain. The amount of blood you see almost always looks many times greater than the actual amount lost.

3. Look at Your Watch or Clock

It is often very helpful if you can tell medical personnel just when the emergency began. Time seems to pass much more quickly in stressful situations. A periodic check of your watch or a clock—if one is easily available—will help you judge time correctly and keep the situation under control.

4. Don't Immediately Rush an Injured Child to the Hospital

Usually, it's better to lose some time waiting for proper emergency transportation of a sick or injured child than to rush the child to the hospital without proper safeguards or handling. The most important thing is to make the child's condition as stable as you can. *Stable* is a term doctors use to mean "in a physical state that is not easily altered." For example, if your child is bleeding, stabilizing the condition would mean stopping the flow of blood.

5. Don't Drive Recklessly

Most injuries, such as badly sprained ankles or deep cuts in which the bleeding has stopped, do not require emergency ambulance transportation. In these situations it is fine to drive to the hospital yourself, but don't speed or drive recklessly. If the injured child is still at an age where he or she needs a car seat, use it! Otherwise, make sure the injured child is safely buckled in by a seat belt. It is better for the child to be uncomfortable for a brief time than to be seriously injured in an accident on the way to the hospital. If possible, have someone sit next to the child.

6. Remember the Telephone

You often can get advice over the telephone to help you stabilize the situation without delay. If a phone is close by, take the time to call your pediatrician or family doctor. You can also *call an emergency room* before going to one. Most emergency rooms have nurses and doctors who are trained to answer questions over the phone. Often, calling an emergency room will save you time and help you quickly begin the proper treatment.

7. Use Common Sense

If you are not sure what to do, use your best guess; it is probably correct. Remember that the least complicated plan is usually right.

8. Trust Your Judgment

You are a mature adult who can handle a difficult situation. Do not second-guess yourself. Do what you think needs to be done.

Cardiopulmonary Resuscitation

There are certain rare situations when a child will stop breathing and his or her heart will stop pumping. These emergencies are almost always caused by accidents of the type that *can be prevented.* (For more details, turn to Part III, "Prevention.")

The more common instances where infants or children might require resuscitation include automobile accidents; accidental overdose of medicines or poisons; near drowning; suffocation caused by a plastic bag, choking on food or a foreign object, or smoke inhalation; a near-miss episode of SIDS (sudden infant death syndrome, formerly called "crib death"); and rare but severe infections of the upper breathing passages.

It is much more common for an adult to need resuscitation than for a child to need it; often an adult needs CPR because of a heart attack, in which the heart stops first and then the lungs fail. A child usually requires resuscitation, because the lungs fail and then the heart stops, as happens in the situations described above. With CPR, which anyone can learn, it's possible for one or two people to keep a victim alive by moving air into the lungs and pumping blood through the heart and around the body's circulatory system.

CPR is a mental and physical skill that must be learned through instruction; it cannot be mastered by reading a book. For this reason I have intentionally omitted from the book any instruction in CPR techniques. The American Red Cross and the American Heart Association both offer courses in CPR. It is usually taught in three to five sessions totaling between 9 and 15 hours of training. Courses are usually available at least once a month and cost between $10 and $35. This life-saving knowledge is clearly worth the price. Your local chapter of either the American Heart Association or the American Red Cross can give you all the details.

CPR saves lives. If you learn the technique, you are much more likely to use it on an adult than on your child, however. The most dangerous time during a heart attack is the first two hours. This is when CPR performed by a relative, neighbor, friend, or stranger passing by could make the difference between life and death before medical personnel arrive.

The CPR technique for infants is different than that used for older children and adults. Make sure that the course you take includes infant resuscitation.

The Emergency Room

Your first contact with a hospital is often the emergency room. While the emergency room serves a vital function, it

can be a very aggravating place for parents. You may have
rushed your child to the hospital for a problem which you are
convinced is a clear emergency and which is probably scaring
the heck out of you; then you *wait* for what can be several
hours to see a doctor.

There are many reasons for this. First of all, most patients
in an emergency room have problems that are not true medical emergencies. These cases clog the emergency room and
slow things down. Another reason for emergency-room de-
lays is that many families do not have doctors (often because
they cannot afford the costs), and they use the emergency
room as they would a clinic or doctor's office. Also, if there
are real emergency cases being treated—say, several people
injured in a motor vehicle accident—you must be prepared to
wait.

There are certain times when emergency rooms are especially busy. Outside of regular working hours and on week-
ends there are fewer doctors in the emergency room. Winter,
during cold and flu season, is a particularly busy time. So are
summer nights during school vacation time; with longer
hours of daylight children stay outside late, and tend to suffer
more injuries, both major and minor. It is surprising, too,
that emergency rooms get very busy on Sunday afternoons
just after the football games on television have ended.

Once in the emergency room, do not expect that your child
will be seen immediately by a doctor. Most emergency rooms
have very experienced nurses who decide the order in which
patients will be seen. For example, cuts are very frightening
and can be quite bloody, but few require immediate attention
from a doctor. If your child has a cut, a nurse will inspect it
and probably clean it and soak the affected area in an iodine
solution for 10 to 20 minutes. Then a doctor will come and
check the cut and put in stitches if the situation warrants their
use. It might be an hour or more before your child is seen by a
doctor, however. But suppose your child is having an asthma
attack and is having difficulty breathing. In this case, the
child will almost always be seen by a doctor within minutes of
reaching the hospital. This is the way an emergency room

works. In each of these examples, the child was given the proper care, at the right time. But "proper care" and "the right time" mean something different in each case.

Once you have decided that your child's problem requires emergency-room treatment, your calm cooperation with the staff there is the best help you can give your child. To make the best use of an emergency room and to reduce the tension you may feel there, follow these guidelines:

1. If you are unsure whether you should bring your child to the hospital, call your doctor. You can also call the emergency room first. Most emergency rooms have experienced nurses who can answer your questions quickly over the phone. You can often begin treatment for your child immediately without having to wait several hours to see a doctor. This is most helpful in cases such as high fever, diarrhea, and vomiting.

2. If your child has had a problem which has not changed for several weeks, such as a rash, do not take him or her to the emergency room. Call your doctor or clinic first.

3. Bring with you any prescription medicines you have been giving your child.

4. Once in the emergency room, do not get angry if your child is not seen immediately by a doctor. Emergency rooms are set up to see patients in the order of the seriousness of their problems, not in the order they came in.

The Hospital

A sick child sometimes has to be admitted to the hospital. This can cause parents to feel both fear and relief at the same time. They are relieved because their child is now under close observation and getting medical care, but they are frightened, or at least upset, because their child is sick and is receiving treatment which they might not understand.

If things are unclear concerning your child's illness or treatment, do not hesitate to ask for more information from the doctors and nurses who are caring for your child. Doctors sometimes forget to use nonmedical language when talking to patients and families, so if you do not understand what the doctor is saying, ask him or her to explain it in clear, nontechnical language. (You'll find a list of medical terms and their definitions in Part IV, "Medical Terms.")

It is important to tell your child as much as possible about the problem and what is going to happen. It is very frightening for a child not to understand what is happening. Too much knowledge is rarely harmful. Perhaps the child has to undergo some painful procedure. Don't say, "It won't hurt," because this will only confuse the child and cause distrust. Be honest. Let children know that it is all right to cry. Tell them that it is important to listen to the doctor and follow instructions.

It is important for sick children to know that they are not bad. Tell your child this. Many young children believe that feeling sick and having painful things done to them is a punishment. When they receive shots or undergo other painful procedures, let them know how very good and brave they are.

Because parents usually want to be with their hospitalized child around the clock, many hospitals provide sleeping facilities for one parent in the child's hospital room.

In the beginning it is proper to be with your child as much as possible. If the hospital stay is going to be more than a few days, however, it is not a good idea to be constantly with the child. You become exhausted and your judgment becomes poor. It is important to avoid this, because at times you will be expected to absorb a great deal of information, learn many new terms and medical principles, and make difficult decisions. You need time for yourself not only to rest and discuss your child's problem, but also to attend to your job responsibilities and other family needs. Having a sick child can be very stressful on your marriage. There may be feelings of anger, guilt, shame, frustration, helplessness, and hopelessness. These issues cannot be handled if you are exhausted.

Nursing care, tests, and other procedures require that parents be separated from their child from time to time. These periodic separations are not harmful to the hospitalized child.

Children requiring care in an intensive care unit, or ICU, receive highly specialized, intensive medical and nursing care which may not allow for prolonged contact with parents. This can be particularly trying for parents. The people on ICU staffs are almost always well attuned to parental concerns and make a great effort to help parents deal with a grave situation.

If there are other children in the family, they will need some special attention as well. Infants and toddlers will do well, but their normal schedule of total care and supervision may require the juggling of baby-sitters, family members, friends, and neighbors. Children of preschool age and older will have to be told in a way they can understand why their brother or sister is in the hospital.

It is very natural for brothers and sisters to be jealous and resentful of the attention given to a sick child. Parents should try to understand these feelings and talk with their well children about them. Children often have fantasies that they may have caused their brother or sister to become ill. For example: a brother who is going to elementary school is very jealous of his new baby sister. In fact, he wishes that he was still the only one around the house. Suddenly one day the baby girl becomes ill and is taken to the hospital. The boy may now believe that he caused her to become ill and he feels scared and guilty. It is very important to tell your other children that they are not responsible for their brother's or sister's illness.

Whenever possible, brothers and sisters should be brought to the hospital to visit the sick infant or child. Different hospitals have different policies regarding sibling visitation, so check with the hospital before arranging a visit.

In spite of worries and fears, the hospital experience does not have to be a terrible one. There are children's books available that explain the experience of being in a hospital. The people working in the hospitals can be counted on to make it as easy as possible.

The hospitalization of a child puts heavy demands on parents. Fortunately, in most situations the experience is bearable. Family members almost always pull together to offer each other aid and comfort.

1. *Bone and Joint Injuries*

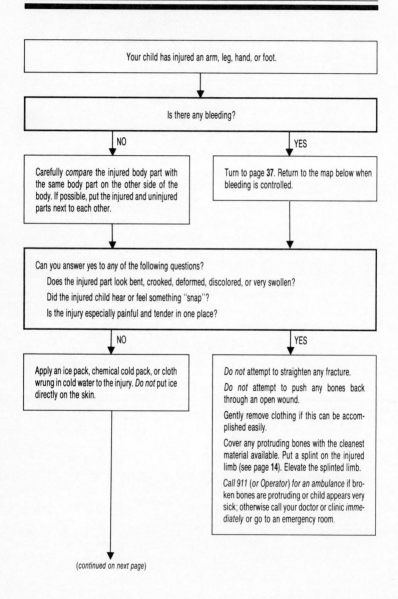

Your child has injured an arm, leg, hand, or foot.

↓

Is there any bleeding?

NO

Carefully *compare* the injured body part with the same body part on the other side of the body. If possible, put the injured and uninjured parts next to each other.

YES

Turn to page **37**. Return to the map below when bleeding is controlled.

↓

Can you answer yes to *any* of the following questions?

Does the injured part look bent, crooked, deformed, discolored, or very swollen?

Did the injured child hear or feel something "snap"?

Is the injury especially painful and tender in one place?

NO

Apply an ice pack, chemical cold pack, or cloth wrung in cold water to the injury. *Do not* put ice directly on the skin.

YES

Do not attempt to straighten any fracture.

Do not attempt to push any bones back through an open wound.

Gently remove clothing if this can be accomplished easily.

Cover any protruding bones with the cleanest material available. Put a splint on the injured limb (see page **14**). Elevate the splinted limb.

Call 911 (or Operator) for an ambulance if broken bones are protruding or child appears very sick; otherwise call your doctor or clinic *immediately* or go to an emergency room.

(continued on next page)

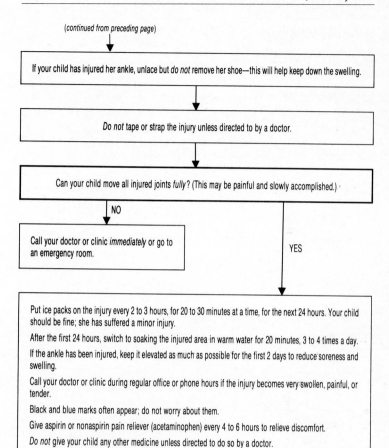

(continued from preceding page)

If your child has injured her ankle, unlace but *do not* remove her shoe—this will help keep down the swelling.

Do not tape or strap the injury unless directed to by a doctor.

Can your child move all injured joints *fully*? (This may be painful and slowly accomplished.)

NO

Call your doctor or clinic *immediately* or go to an emergency room.

YES

Put ice packs on the injury every 2 to 3 hours, for 20 to 30 minutes at a time, for the next 24 hours. Your child should be fine; she has suffered a minor injury.

After the first 24 hours, switch to soaking the injured area in warm water for 20 minutes, 3 to 4 times a day.

If the ankle has been injured, keep it elevated as much as possible for the first 2 days to reduce soreness and swelling.

Call your doctor or clinic during regular office or phone hours if the injury becomes very swollen, painful, or tender.

Black and blue marks often appear; do not worry about them.

Give aspirin or nonaspirin pain reliever (acetaminophen) every 4 to 6 hours to relieve discomfort.

Do not give your child any other medicine unless directed to do so by a doctor.

Have your child rest the injury for at least 2 days, and then begin to reuse the injured body part gradually.

The following instructions are repeated at the end of the book on a tear-out sheet, for quick reference.

Splints and Slings

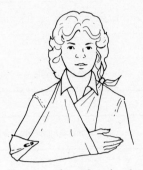

How to make a sling for shoulder, collarbone, or arm injuries.

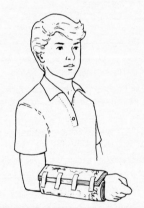

Arm splint using a newspaper or magazine and tape.

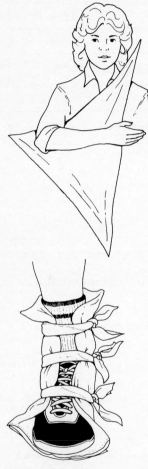

Ankle splint using a pillow and rags.

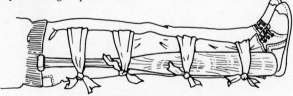

Leg splint using a baseball bat and rags.

More about Bone and Joint Injuries

Bone and joint injuries are very common in childhood. Most of the time these injuries are minor and can be managed properly at home without having to bring the injured child to see a doctor. The map on bone and joint injuries will let you determine confidently when your child has suffered an injury which requires medical attention.

The terminology of limb injuries can be very confusing. The terms commonly used include bruise, strain, sprain, and fracture.

Bruise: A bruise is a lump of the soft tissues under the skin caused by a blow of some sort. There is no break in the skin or bones. The lump is caused by bleeding and irritation of the soft tissues (mostly muscle). The best treatment for a bruise is to apply ice packs for the first 24 hours to reduce the irritation, and heat packs thereafter.

Strain and Sprain: Strains and sprains include any injury that stretches or tears the soft tissues in an arm or leg. The soft tissues include muscles, tendons, and ligaments. Mild or moderate sprains are best treated with rest, elevation, and ice packs. Severe sprains occur when a ligament is completely torn. A ligament is a band of tough tissue, like the gristle in a piece of meat, that connects bones. A severe strain or sprain acts like a fracture and is treated much like a fracture. The ankle is the most commonly sprained joint in the body. Severe strains or sprains should be looked at by a doctor.

Fracture: A fracture is a broken bone. Fractures require prompt medical attention. When the bone protrudes through the skin, the injury is called a *compound fracture;* bleeding is often severe. Compound fractures require hospitalization and surgery.

2. *Breathing Problems*

Breathing problems can be very scary. Try—though it will be difficult—to stay calm and relaxed, because the calmer you are, the calmer your child will be. Symptoms of breathing problems include fast, shallow breathing; shortness of breath when speaking; difficulty breathing in; wheezing; and labored breathing.

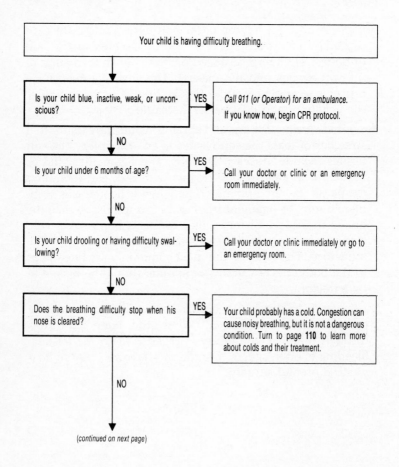

Your child is having difficulty breathing.

Is your child blue, inactive, weak, or unconscious? — **YES** → *Call 911 (or Operator) for an ambulance. If you know how, begin CPR protocol.*

NO

Is your child under 6 months of age? — **YES** → Call your doctor or clinic or an emergency room immediately.

NO

Is your child drooling or having difficulty swallowing? — **YES** → Call your doctor or clinic immediately or go to an emergency room.

NO

Does the breathing difficulty stop when his nose is cleared? — **YES** → Your child probably has a cold. Congestion can cause noisy breathing, but it is not a dangerous condition. Turn to page **110** to learn more about colds and their treatment.

NO

(continued on next page)

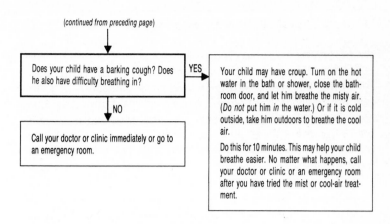

(continued from preceding page)

Does your child have a barking cough? Does he also have difficulty breathing in?

YES → Your child may have croup. Turn on the hot water in the bath or shower, close the bathroom door, and let him breathe the misty air. (*Do not* put him *in* the water.) Or if it is cold outside, take him outdoors to breathe the cool air.

Do this for 10 minutes. This may help your child breathe easier. No matter what happens, call your doctor or clinic or an emergency room after you have tried the mist or cool-air treatment.

NO ↓

Call your doctor or clinic immediately or go to an emergency room.

More about Breathing Problems

Infants and young children have smaller breathing passages and less-developed lungs than adults; therefore, they have breathing problems more often. These breathing problems are usually caused by infections or allergies. Described below are the more common breathing problems seen in infancy and childhood.

CROUP

Croup (rhymes with *soup*) is an infection which causes a barking cough and difficulty breathing in. The cough is often called a *croupy cough*. Croup usually strikes children under 3 years of age. It usually develops gradually after a two- or three-day cold. It often starts at night, accompanied by a mild fever. Croup usually lasts two to three days.

Croup, which usually happens during the late fall and winter, is caused by a germ called a *virus*. Viruses also cause the common cold. In croup the infection is greatest in the breathing passages just below the voice box. This causes the symptoms of barking cough and difficulty breathing in.

Children rarely need to be put in the hospital for croup.

17

However, croup can be serious and has caused death in rare instances. For this reason it is important to notify a doctor when a child first gets croup.

Croup will often respond to misty air, which soothes the breathing passages. Sitting in a steamy bathroom or going out into the cool night air may help stop a bad fit of coughing. A cool-mist humidifier also helps. (Avoid using a hot-mist vaporizer, which can cause burns if it is knocked over.) Antibiotics have no effect against viruses; therefore, they do not help a child with croup.

Breathing faster, turning blue, breathing in with increased difficulty, and showing signs of increased anxiety are all indications that croup is getting worse. If your child should develop any of these problems, call your doctor or go to an emergency room even if your child has already been seen by a doctor.

EPIGLOTTITIS

Epiglottitis (pronounced: eh pee glah *tie* tis), also called *bacterial croup*, is an infection which begins suddenly, generally with a very sore throat, drooling, painful swallowing, high fever, and difficulty breathing in. It can happen at any time of the year. Children 3 to 7 years of age are most susceptible to epiglottitis. It is less common than croup and more dangerous.

Epiglottitis is caused by germs called *bacteria*. The bacteria infect the flap, or epiglottis, that keeps food or drink from going down the windpipe. When the flap gets infected, it swells up and begins to block the windpipe. In severe epiglottitis, the windpipe is totally blocked. This is fatal unless treated.

The doctor will usually get an x-ray to see if a child has epiglottitis. If so, the child will have to stay in the hospital, usually for several days. A breathing tube may be inserted to make sure the breathing passages stay open. Antibiotics are given to kill the bacteria that are causing the problem.

Epiglottitis is a true life-threatening emergency. However,

once the diagnosis is made and the child is in the hospital, the danger is greatly reduced. A child can get epiglottitis only once.

PNEUMONIA

Pneumonia is an infection of the lungs. Usually the lungs are light and filled with air. In pneumonia, solid patches form in the lungs. The condition is usually diagnosed by an x-ray, which shows the infected solid patches. The germs that cause pneumonia include different types of viruses and bacteria.

Pneumonia can take many forms. In its mildest form it may be only a very bad cold. More frequently, pneumonia begins with a mild cold, then over a short period of time fever, cough, and fast breathing develop. The fever may be up to 104° Fahrenheit (40° Celsius). This type of pneumonia is treated at home, except when it occurs in an infant less than 3 or 4 months old. Plenty of clear fluids are important to prevent dehydration, which is a danger in pneumonia because the fever and fast breathing cause the body to lose water.

Doctors often prescribe antibiotics for pneumonia. They are given for a week to 10 days. Aspirin or nonaspirin fever medicine (acetaminophen) will make the child feel more comfortable.

Severe forms of pneumonia will cause difficult breathing, fast breathing, weakness, and a bluish pallor of the skin. Children with severe pneumonia can turn blue because their lungs cannot get enough oxygen. Severe forms of pneumonia require hospitalization. Infants usually have a more difficult time with pneumonia because their lungs are less developed.

In the hospital, children with pneumonia are watched carefully. Extra oxygen is often given either by means of a clear plastic "tent" which covers the hospital crib, or with a face mask. In rare cases children who get very ill with pneumonia need a machine called a *respirator* to help them breathe. Children with pneumonia are usually given fluids and medicines by vein (IV) in the hospital.

Pneumonia is a disease that responds well to treatment.

19

Fortunately, it is now very rarely fatal. Almost all children, including those who have to be hospitalized, fully recover without any long-term problems.

ASTHMA (WHEEZING AND/OR CHRONIC COUGH)

After the common cold, asthma (pronounced: *as* ma) is the most common breathing problem in children. Asthma can take several forms.

Frequent coughing, which is generally worse at night, is a common form. An episode of wheezing and shortness of breath, called an *asthma attack,* is the form of asthma most easily recognized. It often follows what seems to be a two- or three-day "cold," but this is actually the early stage of an asthma attack. Vomiting often occurs with asthma attacks due to an increased amount of mucus, which irritates the throat.

Asthma is caused by the temporary narrowing of small breathing passages, or airways, in the lungs. In people with asthma the airways are very sensitive and easily irritated. Not only do the airways react by narrowing, but they also produce a great deal of mucus. Because the airways are very sensitive, or *reactive*, the medical term for asthma is *reactive airway disease*. Some forms of asthma are caused by allergies, but many people with asthma do not have any allergies.

Most children with asthma have several sensitivities that can trigger attacks. Cigarette smoke is one of the most common triggers; adults should not smoke in the presence of children who have asthma. Other common triggers of asthma attacks include house dust, mites and other insects, pollens, molds, animal hairs, weather changes, air pollution, cooking odors, paint fumes, exercise, and even stress and emotional upset. In rare cases, certain foods, such as fish, nuts, and eggs, can cause asthma attacks. Elimination, as far as possible, of environmental triggers is the cornerstone of asthma treatment.

Children with asthma often have their symptoms during a particular season of the year. Children who are sensitive to molds or house dust and those whose attacks are set off by colds may have their worst symptoms in the winter, especially if they live in houses with forced-air heating. Others may have their worst time during the spring, summer, or fall depending upon the pollens and grasses to which they are sensitive.

Asthma usually begins during younger childhood, but it can start at any age from infancy to adulthood. An older child who previously had no evidence of asthma may develop a chronic cough, following a bad cold, which never seems to go away. This is evidence that the airways have become sensitive. The infection which caused the cold was the triggering event.

Asthma often runs in families where there is a medical history of allergies. Hay fever and eczema are other allergic diseases that can occur in children or families with a history of asthma. (Eczema is a type of skin rash; see page 186.)

An acute asthma attack is an emergency that requires medical attention. Cough medicine, decongestants, and cold remedies have no place in the treatment of acute asthma attacks. Antibiotics are rarely helpful; they only kill bacteria, and bacterial infections hardly ever trigger attacks. Colds can trigger asthma attacks, but colds are caused by viruses, and viruses are not killed by antibiotics.

There are specific medicines which a doctor can prescribe that work well against asthma. The quickest-acting medicines are epinephrine, which is given under the skin as a shot, and medicines that are inhaled, called *aerosols*. Epinephrine takes about 20 minutes to act, and the person may feel shaky and jittery after receiving the injection. The relieving effect of epinephrine is brief. Another medicine used for asthma, theophylline, is longer-acting. It is usually taken by mouth in the form of liquid, syrup, tablets, or capsules. There are many different brands of theophylline; a few of them are Slophyllin,® Somophyllin,® Quibron,® and Theodur®. There are also many different medications which can be inhaled into the lungs in aerosol form. Extra oxygen is usually given to children who are hospitalized with asthma. Steroids are very useful in more severe attacks; they make the theophylline work better. Steroids are safe when used for short periods of time.

The medicines used to treat asthma are more effective the earlier they are started. Parents should learn from experience to recognize the early symptoms of an attack and start the medicine at that point. Some children get medicine only during the season of the year when their symptoms appear.

Children can become dehydrated during asthma attacks, so it is important to encourage the intake of fluids. They should be clear fluids; water and apple juice are particularly good. (See Chapter 23, "Diarrhea," and Chapter 41, "Vomiting," for more information about dehydration and clear fluids.) Solid foods also should not be eaten during an asthma attack because they can cause choking.

Asthma has a wide range of severity. Some children experience frequent attacks and have to be on medicine all the time. Other children have few attacks and need medicine only a couple of times a year. Many children with asthma never have to be hospitalized. Others may require hospitalization from time to time.

Parents must exercise careful judgment once their child has been diagnosed as having asthma. It's important to know when to start and when to stop the theophylline or aerosol medication. In general, you should call your doctor when you have any questions or concerns and when your child exhibits any of these symptoms:

Persistent coughing and/or wheezing which does not respond to medication

Repeated vomiting

Difficulty speaking because of shortness of breath

Difficulty sleeping because of wheezing, labored breathing, or persistent coughing

Upset stomach, loss of appetite, vomiting, headaches, jumpiness, or hyperactivity (all side effects of theophylline)

It is difficult to predict whether a specific child will outgrow his or her asthma. Some children continue to have asthma in the same form as adults; some children get worse. But many children do outgrow it. Great advances have been made recently in the treatment of asthma. It is now rarely life-threatening. Most children respond well to their medicines and live full and active lives.

WHEEZING IN INFANTS

Infants less than 2 years old may develop a certain type of breathing problem during winter months. It is called *bronchiolitis* (pronounced: bronk ee o *lie* tis). This condition usually starts after an infant has had a runny nose for a day or two. Rapid breathing, coughing, and wheezing are the main features.

The usual cause of bronchiolitis is an infection with a type of virus, called *RSV* for short, that involves the coverings of small airways in infants' lungs.

Bronchiolitis is usually not very serious. Many infants continue to eat and play normally while the illness runs its course. Infants with bronchiolitis must be seen by a doctor, however, because a few will need to be put into the hospital. Hospital treatment usually consists of close observation while extra oxygen is given to the infant by means of a clear plastic oxygen tent that goes over the hospital crib. Bronchiolitis usually lasts only several days.

SUDDEN INFANT DEATH SYNDROME (SIDS)

Sudden infant death syndrome (SIDS) is defined as the sudden, unexpected, death of any infant that remains unexplained even after an autopsy. Other terms used for SIDS include *cot death* and *crib death*.

While there have been many theories proposed, the cause of SIDS remains unknown. Nine out of ten cases occur during the first 6 months of life; essentially, SIDS never occurs over the age of 12 months. It always occurs during sleep and is silent. Usually, an infant struck with SIDS has been entirely healthy before the event; some infants may have had mild colds just before they died. The risk of SIDS is greater in infants whose families have already had a SIDS event.

Families who have suffered the loss of a child to SIDS should receive counseling from specially trained individuals. There is a network of support groups made up of parents who have suffered the loss of a child from SIDS. The National Sudden Infant Death Foundation, Inc., may be of help; the address is 8240 Professional Place, Suite 205, Landover, MD 20785, and the telephone number is 1-800-221-SIDS.

NEAR-MISS SIDS

A near-miss SIDS event is a frightening episode in which an infant is found to be limp, blue, and not breathing. The infant recovers following vigorous stimulation or resuscitation. Infants who experience near-miss SIDS events should always be admitted to the hospital for extensive medical testing, as they are at increased risk for SIDS.

APNEA

Apnea is a temporary pause in breathing. Apnea can be normal or abnormal depending on its frequency and duration. An *apnea monitor* is a device that detects pauses in breathing during sleep. An alarm sounds when the infant has a pause in breathing that is too long or when the heart rate drops too low. Those placed on apnea monitors include certain premature infants, infants who have suffered near-miss SIDS events, and infants who have had an older brother or sister die from SIDS.

3. *Burns*

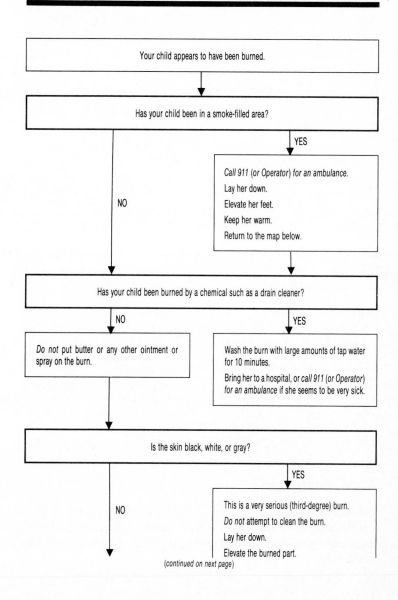

Your child appears to have been burned.

Has your child been in a smoke-filled area?

YES

Call 911 (or Operator) for an ambulance.
Lay her down.
Elevate her feet.
Keep her warm.
Return to the map below.

NO

Has your child been burned by a chemical such as a drain cleaner?

NO

Do not put butter or any other ointment or spray on the burn.

YES

Wash the burn with large amounts of tap water for 10 minutes.
Bring her to a hospital, or *call 911 (or Operator) for an ambulance* if she seems to be very sick.

Is the skin black, white, or gray?

NO

YES

This is a very serious (third-degree) burn.
Do not attempt to clean the burn.
Lay her down.
Elevate the burned part.

(continued on next page)

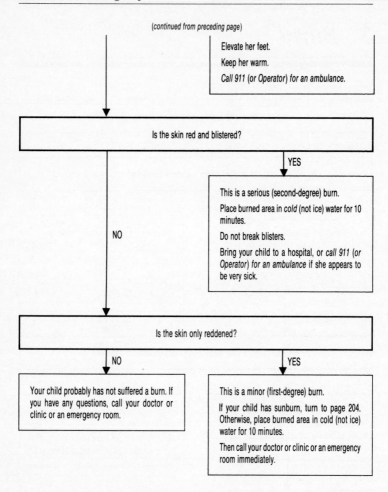

(continued from preceding page)

Elevate her feet.

Keep her warm.

Call 911 (or Operator) for an ambulance.

Is the skin red and blistered?

YES

This is a serious (second-degree) burn.

Place burned area in *cold* (not ice) water for 10 minutes.

Do not break blisters.

Bring your child to a hospital, or *call 911 (or Operator) for an ambulance* if she appears to be very sick.

NO

Is the skin only reddened?

NO

Your child probably has not suffered a burn. If you have any questions, call your doctor or clinic or an emergency room.

YES

This is a minor (first-degree) burn.

If your child has sunburn, turn to page 204. Otherwise, place burned area in cold (not ice) water for 10 minutes.

Then call your doctor or clinic or an emergency room immediately.

More about Burns

Burns rank high among the causes of severe injury during childhood. They are almost always preventable; see the list of measures you can take to prevent burns given in Part III, "Prevention."

Young children and infants burn more easily and more severely than adults do because they have such very thin skin. The common causes of burns include scalds, which often occur when a toddler pulls a pot or pan containing a hot liquid off the stove; contact burns from stoves, irons, and hot kitchen utensils; chemical burns from strong acidic or alkaline substances such as drain cleaners; electrical burns (see Chapter 8, "Electrical Injuries"); and flame burns, which often result from burning clothing.

Home Burn Care

All burns, except for small, minor (first-degree) burns, should be evaluated by a physician. The common practice of covering a burn with butter or some other ointment or spray is *not a good idea;* it only serves to complicate the burn, making infection more likely. Cooling the skin with cold water is the best initial treatment for all burns. It is most important to keep a burn dressing *clean* and *dry.* The classification of burns is described on the burn map.

Hospitalization

Less severe burns may require frequent visits to the doctor for dressing changes; some may require hospitalization. Severe burns require intensive treatment, which is often given in special burn units. The problems involved with severe burns include infection, fluid imbalance, breathing difficulty, pain, emotional problems, cosmetic problems, and long-term disability. Children with severe burns spend an average of two months in the hospital. This can be particularly difficult for both the child and the family.

Burns take a long time to heal: at least two weeks for even second-degree burns, months for third-degree burns. Severe burns form scar tissue which tightens and contracts over time. These contractures can be particularly disabling, especially when the hands are involved. Multiple surgical operations over several years may be required.

Smoke Inhalation

Smoke inhalation can cause severe, life-threatening injury to the lungs. This injury can take 24 to 48 hours to develop. Anyone exposed to a smoky fire should be seen by a physician no matter how well they appear to be following the exposure.

A Word about Child Abuse

Child abuse often involves burns, especially cigarette burns. There may be one or more of these round, quarter-inch burns. Scalding with boiling water is another type of burn commonly inflicted on children.

If you suspect child abuse or are uncertain about the circumstances surrounding a burn your child has received, turn to Chapter 18, "Child Abuse," where this topic is dealt with in further detail.

4. *Choking*

The following instructions are repeated at the end of the book on a tear-out sheet which can be placed in the kitchen, perhaps taped to the refrigerator.

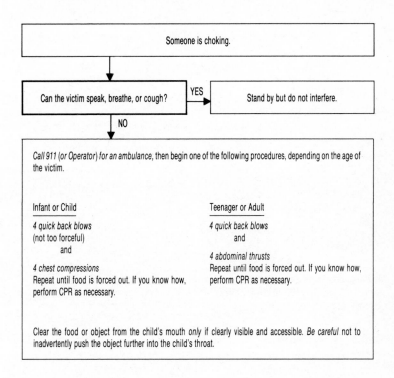

Someone is choking.

Can the victim speak, breathe, or cough? **YES** → Stand by but do not interfere.

NO

Call 911 (or Operator) for an ambulance, then begin one of the following procedures, depending on the age of the victim.

Infant or Child

4 quick back blows
(not too forceful)
        and

4 chest compressions
Repeat until food is forced out. If you know how, perform CPR as necessary.

Teenager or Adult

4 quick back blows
        and

4 abdominal thrusts
Repeat until food is forced out. If you know how, perform CPR as necessary.

Clear the food or object from the child's mouth *only* if clearly visible and accessible. *Be careful* not to inadvertently push the object further into the child's throat.

First Aid for Someone Who Is Choking

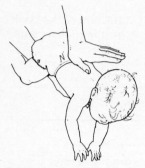

Infant receiving back blows.

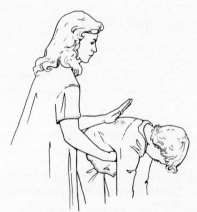

Child receiving back blows.

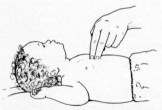

Infant receiving chest compressions. (*Note:* Only two fingers are used.)

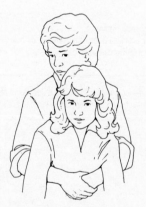

Child receiving abdominal thrusts. (*Note:* Direction of thrust is an inward and upward motion.)

More about Choking

Choking is the most common cause of accidental death in children under 6 years of age. Peanuts, corn, and safety pins are some of the things that commonly cause choking in children. As we know, infants and young children will put everything and anything into their mouths, and often they swallow these objects harmlessly. That is, the object goes down the food tube and enters the stomach. But sometimes the object enters and blocks the windpipe. Coughing is the body's natural way of clearing the windpipe, but the child may not be able to cough. Such a blockage of the windpipe will be fatal unless it is relieved quickly.

Poor chewing is another cause of choking. Children do not chew very well until they are around 4 or 5 years old. That is why it is so important to feed young children only soft foods and foods chopped up into small pieces.

Prevention of Choking

- *Never* leave small objects within an infant's or small child's reach even for a moment.

- *Never* feed your infant or young child *large* or *hard pieces of food*, especially hard candy or large pieces of meat.

- *Never* feed *peanuts, bacon, or popcorn* to your child until he or she is 6 or 7 years old. Peanuts are very slippery and can easily pass into a child's windpipe. Bacon breaks into small slivers, which also can easily travel into the lungs. Popcorn is very light and can be sucked into a child's lungs.

- *Gum* should not be given to children under 6 or 7 years of age.

- *Never* give your child *uninflated balloons* to play with. These can be very dangerous, because they can easily be sucked down the windpipe.

5. Convulsions (Seizures)

Seizures can be very frightening to watch. The signs include shaking, stiffening, jerking, and arching of the back. Your child may not be able to answer you, but remember that he is not in pain. Try to stay calm.

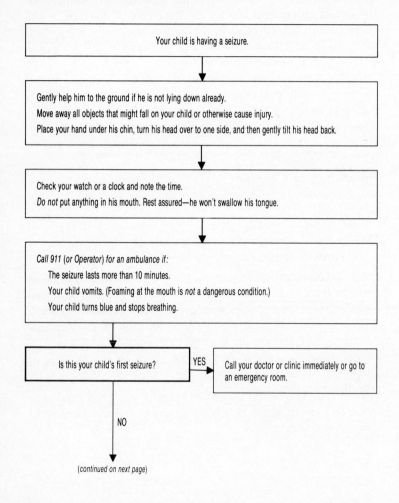

Your child is having a seizure.

Gently help him to the ground if he is not lying down already.

Move away all objects that might fall on your child or otherwise cause injury.

Place your hand under his chin, turn his head over to one side, and then gently tilt his head back.

Check your watch or a clock and note the time.

Do not put anything in his mouth. Rest assured—he won't swallow his tongue.

Call 911 (or Operator) for an ambulance if:

The seizure lasts more than 10 minutes.

Your child vomits. (Foaming at the mouth is *not* a dangerous condition.)

Your child turns blue and stops breathing.

Is this your child's first seizure? —YES→ Call your doctor or clinic immediately or go to an emergency room.

NO

(continued on next page)

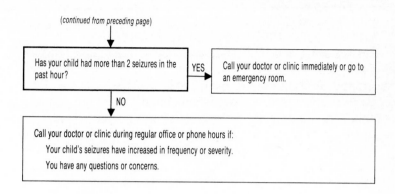

(continued from preceding page)

Has your child had more than 2 seizures in the past hour? **YES** → Call your doctor or clinic immediately or go to an emergency room.

NO

Call your doctor or clinic during regular office or phone hours if:

Your child's seizures have increased in frequency or severity.

You have any questions or concerns.

More about Seizures

A seizure is caused by the brain sending a burst of abnormal signals. The brain contains billions of cells, so small that they can be seen only with a microscope. Each of these cells produces a very small amount of electricity. A seizure occurs when many cells fire at once in a disordered way.

Convulsions take many forms. As mentioned, there may be shaking, stiffening, jerking, or arching of the back. The eyes may roll to expose the white part, or they may turn to one side. A child may cry out at the beginning of a convulsion. The cry is caused not by pain but by air being forced out through the voice box as the muscles of the chest and belly contract. There may be foaming at the mouth and loud gurgling noises during the seizure. The child may wet his pants or have a bowel movement.

The medical term for a shaking or jerking seizure that involves the arms and legs is *grand mal seizure*. After a grand mal seizure a child will sleep, usually quite deeply, for a period of time anywhere from a half hour to several hours. This sleepy phase is not part of the seizure itself and should not be included in calculating the duration of the seizure. The medical term for this phase is the *postictal* (pronounced: post *ick* tel) *phase*.

A seizure which involves jerking or shaking is sometimes

termed a *convulsion*. Not all seizures involve jerking or shaking. Seizures can also take the form of brief staring or blinking spells during which the child cannot respond to questions. In some seizures the child loses his posture and falls to the ground. A child cannot make a seizure happen. Similarly, a parent cannot cause a seizure to happen—by punishing a child, for example.

Do not stick *anything* into the mouth of a person having a seizure, especially your fingers. Whatever you may have heard, it's impossible to "swallow your tongue" and suffocate during a convulsion. It is true that during a seizure a person can bite and cut his tongue, but these cuts usually are not deep. More harm can come from an object placed in the mouth which can cut or choke the person or be swallowed.

Seizures do not cause brain damage. The greatest danger from a seizure is that it may occur when the child is engaged in some potentially dangerous activity—swimming, for example. A few other dangerous problems can occur with seizures. Vomiting during or at the end of a seizure can interfere with breathing if food particles get into the breathing passages. This is why you are instructed to lay the child down and turn his head to one side during a seizure; this helps keep vomited material out of the breathing passages. A seizure that causes breathing to stop requires immediate medical attention. Lastly, a seizure that lasts longer than 10 minutes can be dangerous because it may be difficult to stop. Fortunately, all of these problems are very rare.

You may be very frightened the first time you see a child having a convulsion. The child appears to be in pain, yet he does not feel any pain during the event. His muscles may be sore afterward, and he may have a headache.

It may be hard for you to do, but try to stay calm, cool, and collected.

Epilepsy

The term *epilepsy* means repeated seizures that occur without fever. (Seizures that occur with fever are discussed in the next section.) Unfortunately, some people are still prejudiced or ignorant about seizures and epilepsy. They should understand that a person with epilepsy does not have brain damage, retardation, mental illness, a nervous disorder, or a personality problem.

Seizure disorder is a medical term that many prefer to use instead of *epilepsy*. It means the same thing. This condition can occur for many different reasons. It can accompany other medical problems, some of which are serious, but just as often it occurs in intelligent children who are otherwise normal and healthy. Why it happens in these otherwise normal and healthy children is still not understood. There are many medicines available now that work well in preventing seizures. They are called *anticonvulsants.*

Seizures are often diagnosed with the help of an electroencephalogram, or EEG. This is also called a *brain wave test.* It is a painless test that measures the electric activity of the brain by means of electrodes, small pieces of metal that are taped or temporarily glued to the scalp. Infants and young children may be given medicine to make them sleepy before an EEG.

For many children and families the emotional impact of epilepsy is far greater than the physical danger. Children may feel "different" or embarrassed because they have seizures. Teenagers often resent the loss of control over their bodies which seizures cause. They also do not like having to take the few precautions necessary or taking their daily doses of medicine.

Driving an automobile may be a problem for someone who has seizures. This issue is particularly difficult for teenagers. While laws vary from state to state, as a general rule, an individual must be seizure-free at least 1 to 2 years, either on or off medication, before he is eligible to apply for a license. While the temptation to hide the fact of seizures is great, the ramifications of a seizure-related car accident can be devastating.

Parents of epileptic children will have to deal with many issues and may need the support and advice of their doctors.

There are also support groups made up of parents of epileptic children.

It is best to raise a child with epilepsy in a normal manner. Participation in regular sports activity should be encouraged—with a few exceptions. These include high climbing and using climbing ropes, using a trampoline, and swimming alone (something no one should do anyway). There are some restrictions, but most children with seizures can lead full, active lives. Most children who are otherwise healthy outgrow seizures as they become young adults.

SEIZURES WITH FEVER (FEBRILE SEIZURES)

It is not uncommon for healthy children between 3 months and 6 years of age to have seizures with fever. These are called *febrile seizures*. They happen because children have less developed brains, in which fever may trigger a seizure. Febrile seizures do not cause brain damage.

The first time an infant or child has a febrile seizure, he must be seen by a doctor. This is to make sure that there is no other problem present, especially in children less than 2 years old. Once a child has had a febrile seizure, there is about a fifty-fifty chance that the child will have more attacks. The best way to treat febrile seizures is to give nonaspirin fever medicine (acetaminophen) every four hours whenever fever develops. Anticonvulsant medication, which must be taken continually, is sometimes necessary.

Seizures of this type only slightly increase the risk that a child will develop epilepsy. An otherwise normal child who has experienced an uncomplicated febrile seizure has only 2 chances in 100 (2 percent) of getting epilepsy. Children outgrow febrile seizures by 6 years of age.

6. Cuts and Bleeding

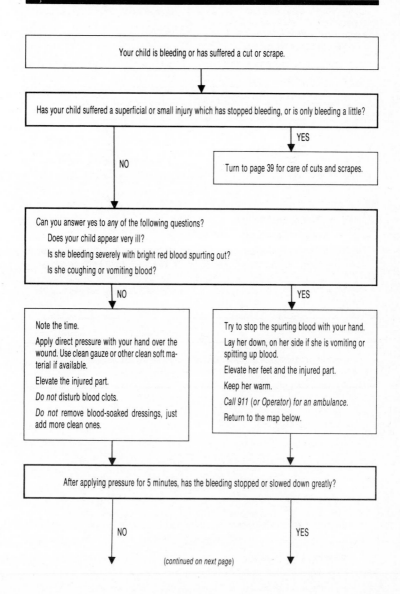

Your child is bleeding or has suffered a cut or scrape.

Has your child suffered a superficial or small injury which has stopped bleeding, or is only bleeding a little?

YES

NO

Turn to page 39 for care of cuts and scrapes.

Can you answer yes to *any* of the following questions?

Does your child appear very ill?

Is she bleeding severely with bright red blood spurting out?

Is she coughing or vomiting blood?

NO

YES

Note the time.

Apply direct pressure with your hand over the wound. Use clean gauze or other clean soft material if available.

Elevate the injured part.

Do not disturb blood clots.

Do not remove blood-soaked dressings, just add more clean ones.

Try to stop the spurting blood with your hand.

Lay her down, on her side if she is vomiting or spitting up blood.

Elevate her feet and the injured part.

Keep her warm.

Call 911 (or Operator) for an ambulance.

Return to the map below.

After applying pressure for 5 minutes, has the bleeding stopped or slowed down greatly?

NO

YES

(continued on next page)

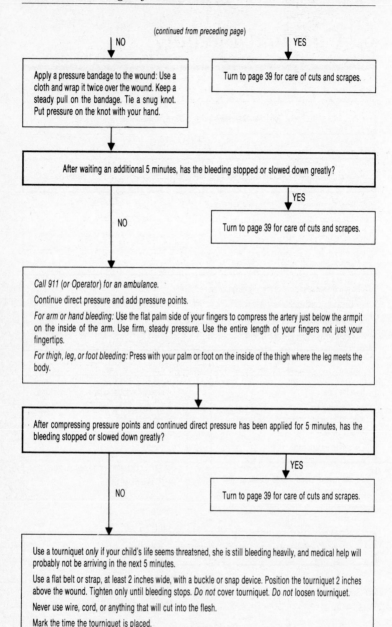

(continued from preceding page)

↓ NO   ↓ YES

Apply a pressure bandage to the wound: Use a cloth and wrap it twice over the wound. Keep a steady pull on the bandage. Tie a snug knot. Put pressure on the knot with your hand.

Turn to page 39 for care of cuts and scrapes.

After waiting an additional 5 minutes, has the bleeding stopped or slowed down greatly?

↓ YES

Turn to page 39 for care of cuts and scrapes.

NO

Call 911 (or Operator) for an ambulance.

Continue direct pressure and add pressure points.

For arm or hand bleeding: Use the flat palm side of your fingers to compress the artery just below the armpit on the inside of the arm. Use firm, steady pressure. Use the entire length of your fingers not just your fingertips.

For thigh, leg, or foot bleeding: Press with your palm or foot on the inside of the thigh where the leg meets the body.

After compressing pressure points and continued direct pressure has been applied for 5 minutes, has the bleeding stopped or slowed down greatly?

↓ YES

Turn to page 39 for care of cuts and scrapes.

NO

Use a tourniquet *only* if your child's life seems threatened, she is still bleeding heavily, and medical help will probably not be arriving in the next 5 minutes.

Use a flat belt or strap, at least 2 inches wide, with a buckle or snap device. Position the tourniquet 2 inches above the wound. Tighten only until bleeding stops. *Do not* cover tourniquet. *Do not* loosen tourniquet.

Never use wire, cord, or anything that will cut into the flesh.

Mark the time the tourniquet is placed.

Care of Cuts and Scrapes

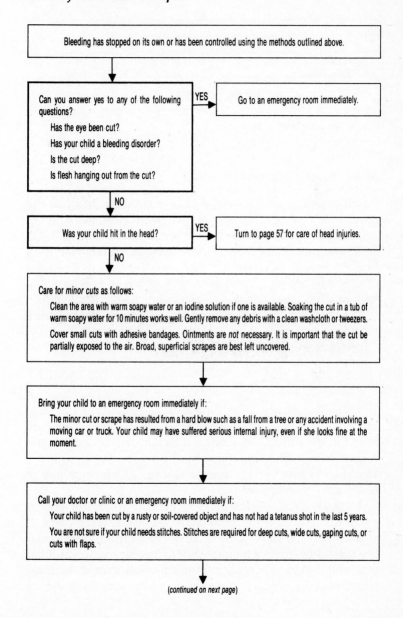

Bleeding has stopped on its own or has been controlled using the methods outlined above.

Can you answer yes to *any* of the following questions?

Has the eye been cut?

Has your child a bleeding disorder?

Is the cut deep?

Is flesh hanging out from the cut?

YES → Go to an emergency room immediately.

NO

Was your child hit in the head? **YES** → Turn to page 57 for care of head injuries.

NO

Care for *minor cuts* as follows:

Clean the area with warm soapy water or an iodine solution if one is available. Soaking the cut in a tub of warm soapy water for 10 minutes works well. Gently remove any debris with a clean washcloth or tweezers.

Cover small cuts with adhesive bandages. Ointments are *not* necessary. It is important that the cut be partially exposed to the air. Broad, superficial scrapes are best left uncovered.

Bring your child to an emergency room immediately if:

The minor cut or scrape has resulted from a hard blow such as a fall from a tree or any accident involving a moving car or truck. Your child may have suffered serious internal injury, even if she looks fine at the moment.

Call your doctor or clinic or an emergency room immediately if:

Your child has been cut by a rusty or soil-covered object and has not had a tetanus shot in the last 5 years.

You are not sure if your child needs stitches. Stitches are required for deep cuts, wide cuts, gaping cuts, or cuts with flaps.

(continued on next page)

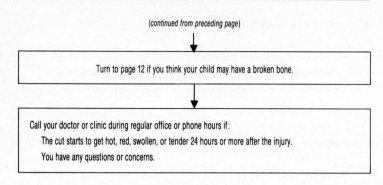

Turn to page 12 if you think your child may have a broken bone.

Call your doctor or clinic during regular office or phone hours if:
    The cut starts to get hot, red, swollen, or tender 24 hours or more after the injury.
    You have any questions or concerns.

More about Cuts and Bleeding

Minor cuts and scrapes are part of childhood. Most of the time these injuries can be handled easily at home. The appearance of blood can be quite frightening but remember, a small amount of blood can appear to be a very large amount. Just a teaspoon of blood dripped onto the shirt of a toddler can look terrifying. Try to stay calm. The cut or scrape will look much better once it is cleaned and the bleeding stops.

The maps on the preceding pages will direct you in caring for minor as well as more serious cuts and wounds.

A Word about Tetanus

Tetanus, or lockjaw, is an illness caused by a type of germ, called a *bacterium*. The specific bacteria that cause tetanus are found in the ground. A tetanus infection can develop in any wound from a dirty object that has been lying on the ground. The illness causes severe muscle spasms which begin one to seven days after the injury.

Tetanus immunization gives 99 percent protection against a tetanus infection; the protection lasts for several years. If your child has missed some or all of her immunization shots, she should be given a tetanus shot following any wound that breaks the skin. Thereafter, immunization should be completed as soon as possible according to the doctor's or clinic's advice. Your child will need to get a booster tetanus shot following a clean, minor wound only if she has not had a tetanus shot within 10 years. For other, more serious, wounds, a booster shot will be needed only if she has not had a tetanus shot within 5 years.

Internal Bleeding

Bleeding in the chest or abdominal cavities usually results from hard blows. Internal bleeding is often not visible, and it can be extremely dangerous, even fatal at times. The early signs of internal bleeding can be very slight, however. Any time a child suffers a hard blow, such as being hit by a car or falling from a significant height, it is important to bring her to the doctor or an emergency room no matter how good she looks after the injury. If too much blood is lost from internal bleeding, the brain and other vital organs will be compromised and shock will follow.

Shock is the medical term for severely low blood pressure. Severe blood loss from any source can cause shock. The symptoms include pallor, weakness, dizziness, faintness, cold and clammy skin, and weak and rapid pulse. Eventually the injured person passes out. The medical term *shock* does not mean a fainting spell, severe fright, or being startled.

7. *Drowning*

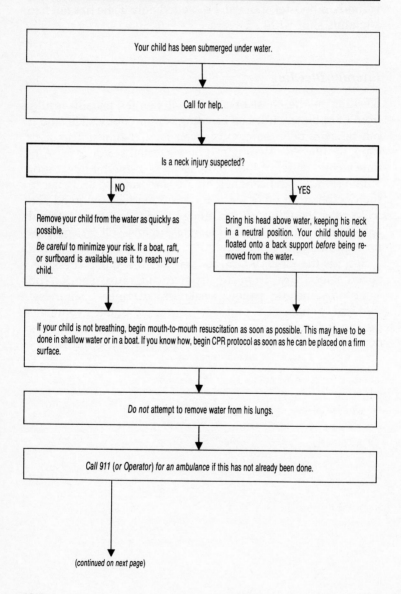

Your child has been submerged under water.

↓

Call for help.

↓

Is a neck injury suspected?

NO ← → **YES**

Remove your child from the water as quickly as possible. *Be careful* to minimize your risk. If a boat, raft, or surfboard is available, use it to reach your child.	Bring his head above water, keeping his neck in a neutral position. Your child should be floated onto a back support *before* being removed from the water.

↓

If your child is not breathing, begin mouth-to-mouth resuscitation as soon as possible. This may have to be done in shallow water or in a boat. If you know how, begin CPR protocol as soon as he can be placed on a firm surface.

↓

Do not attempt to remove water from his lungs.

↓

Call 911 (or Operator) for an ambulance if this has not already been done.

↓

(continued on next page)

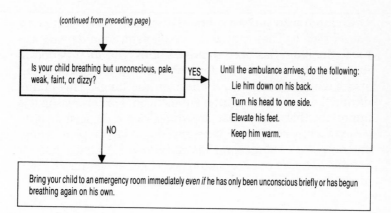

(continued from preceding page)

Is your child breathing but unconscious, pale, weak, faint, or dizzy? — **YES** → Until the ambulance arrives, do the following:
Lie him down on his back.
Turn his head to one side.
Elevate his feet.
Keep him warm.

NO ↓

Bring your child to an emergency room immediately *even if* he has only been unconscious briefly or has begun breathing again on his own.

More about Drowning

Drowning is one of the leading causes of death among children and teenagers in the United States. Most drownings are preventable accidents that occur in fresh water a few feet from safety. Prevention is discussed in detail in the next section, "Water Safety."

Drownings occur year-round, but they peak during the summer months. Community swimming pools were once the leading site of drownings; now, drownings occur more commonly in backyard pools, which are less likely to be supervised and properly enclosed.

Infants and young children are more likely to drown in unprotected ponds or backyard swimming pools, while unattended in the bathtub, or after a fall through ice. Most older children drown while swimming, boating, diving, or participating in some other water sport without proper supervision or experience. Alcohol or drug abuse is associated with certain instances of drowning in teenagers and adults.

Drowning is a form of *suffocation,* a condition in which oxygen is prevented from reaching the lungs and passing into the bloodstream. Drowning causes suffocation either by filling the lungs with water or by causing the voice box in the throat to shut tight in spasm.

Children who survive submersion in water have suffered a *near drowning*. They may have permanent brain damage because the brain has been deprived of oxygen for a period of time, usually exceeding a few minutes. Near drowning can also have a serious *delayed* effect on the lungs. This occurs during the first 24 hours after submersion. For this reason it is important that every near-drowning victim be seen *immediately* by a physician even if he appears to be completely fine, and even if the submersion has been brief. Hospitalization for at least 24 hours of observation is recommended for all near-drowning victims.

Water Safety

SWIMMING SAFETY

- **Never swim alone.** Make sure your children are *always supervised* by a responsible adult or older teenager. Toddlers are notorious for straying off. They need particularly close supervision.

- Do not swim when you are overtired or overheated, after you have been drinking alcohol, or after you have eaten a particularly large meal. It is safe to let your child swim after a light meal or snack.

- Do not overestimate your ability to swim. Ocean currents can be deceptive. Accurately judging distance over water is very difficult.

- Do not swim in unfamiliar places, since they may contain hazards such as dangerous currents, deep holes, or debris.

- Before diving into the water, especially into a pool you have never been in before, *check to make sure it is deep enough.* Pools can look much deeper than they actually are. Many people have injured themselves tragically by diving head first into shallow pools. This can result in total paralysis from the neck down.

- Make sure all family members are taught how to float and swim at the earliest age possible. It is fine to bring young infants and toddlers into the water with you if it is warm water. Organized swimming instruction is not advisable before the age of 3 years, however, because before this time a child's head is disproportionately large and he cannot hold it out of the water. A child of at least 3 years of age who can hold his breath on command is ready to learn to swim. Even young children who have been taught to swim cannot be considered water-safe; they cannot be relied upon to retain their swimming skills in an emergency. They can inhale enough water in a few brief moments to cause seizures, coma, or death. There is no substitute for adequate supervision and safeguards.

- Make sure all family members are taught basic water safety and first-aid skills. Instruction in swimming, scuba diving, and waterskiing should be obtained only from qualified instructors.

- Everyone should stay out of the water during electrical storms.

- A playful atmosphere around water is fine, but wild and reckless behavior should not be tolerated. Games involving false alarms such as "calling for help" should never be permitted.

POOL SAFETY

- Make sure your pool is properly fenced in. This applies to *any* pool, including portable, above-ground pools. Fences should be between 4 and 6 feet high and have self-locking latches. Check your local ordinance for other rules.

- Keep the barrier around your pool clear of objects which could enable a child to climb into the pool area.

- Diving boards should be used only in water that is deep enough. A depth of 8½ feet (2.6 meters) may be too shallow for a skilled diver.

- Paint numbers on the pool edge indicating depth at various points.

- Use a ladder with steps at least 3 inches wide made of nonslip material.
- Pool slides are very dangerous and should be avoided.
- Essential first-aid equipment and rescue devices should be ready at the pool.
- Allow no tricycles, bicycles, wagons, glass objects, or electric appliances at poolside.
- Place a tamper-proof cover over the pool when it is unattended.

BOATING SAFETY

- The adult in charge of a boat should be fully competent in its use. The boat must be seaworthy; ask the Coast Guard Auxiliary to make a courtesy inspection of it if you are not sure.
- Check weather reports before going out on the water.
- Do not overload the boat.
- At least one adult swimmer should be present for each nonswimming child. The adults should know which child they are responsible for.
- Do not allow standing in small boats.
- *Always wear a life jacket* or other flotation device when boating. There should be a life jacket of proper size for every person on board.

Finally, you should make sure that your community has an active program of public education in water safety.

8. *Electrical Injuries*

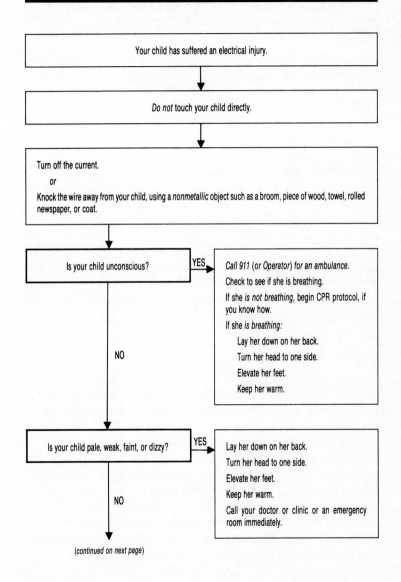

Your child has suffered an electrical injury.

Do not touch your child directly.

Turn off the current.

    or

Knock the wire away from your child, using a *nonmetallic* object such as a broom, piece of wood, towel, rolled newspaper, or coat.

Is your child unconscious? **YES**

Call 911 (or Operator) for an ambulance.

Check to see if she is breathing.

If she *is not breathing*, begin CPR protocol, if you know how.

If she *is breathing:*

    Lay her down on her back.

    Turn her head to one side.

    Elevate her feet.

    Keep her warm.

NO

Is your child pale, weak, faint, or dizzy? **YES**

Lay her down on her back.

Turn her head to one side.

Elevate her feet.

Keep her warm.

Call your doctor or clinic or an emergency room immediately.

NO

(continued on next page)

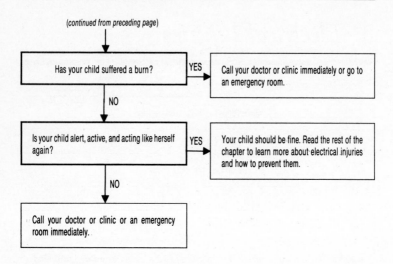

More about Electrical Injuries

Electrical shocks and burns are serious injuries which are almost always preventable. They may result from low-voltage lines in the home, high-voltage transmission lines, and—in rare instances—lightning.

ELECTRICAL BURNS

Electrical burns usually are caused by low-voltage household current. Toddlers and preschoolers often sustain electrical burns of the mouth from biting an electric cord, or burns of the fingertips from sticking a metal object into an electric outlet. Mouth burns can cause profuse bleeding.

High-voltage injuries are seen typically in older children and teenagers who play on electrified rail lines or in transformer stations. These burns tend to be deep within muscles and may cause deceptively little skin damage; only after several days does the full extent of the damage to the muscles become obvious. High-voltage current often leaves entrance and exit burns. It can cause loss of limbs or death.

Any child who has suffered an electrical burn should be seen immediately by a doctor. Hospitalization is often necessary.

ELECTRICAL SHOCKS

If enough electric current passes through the body, you can be knocked unconscious due to either a sudden arrest of breathing or abnormal beating of the heart. High-voltage current is more dangerous than low-voltage current in this regard. Also, alternating current (AC) is more likely to affect the heart than is direct current (DC). Alternating current is the type found in homes; direct current is the type produced by batteries.

Prevention of Electrical Injuries

- If you have an infant or young child, make sure all electric outlets are covered by safety caps.
- As your infant begins to crawl and explore, make sure all electric cords are out of biting range.
- Educate older children to the dangers of high-power lines, high-voltage transformer stations, and the "third rail" of electrified train tracks.
- Always make sure that electric appliances are properly installed. This is particularly important for appliances that require heavy-duty lines, such as stoves, washers, and driers.
- Do not overload household lines with multiple plugs, and never place a penny under a "blown" fuse.

9. *Eye Injuries*

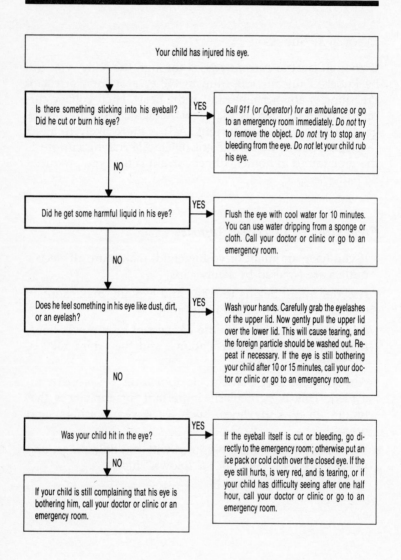

Your child has injured his eye.

Is there something sticking into his eyeball? Did he cut or burn his eye?

YES → *Call 911 (or Operator) for an ambulance* or go to an emergency room immediately. *Do not* try to remove the object. *Do not* try to stop any bleeding from the eye. *Do not* let your child rub his eye.

NO ↓

Did he get some harmful liquid in his eye?

YES → Flush the eye with cool water for 10 minutes. You can use water dripping from a sponge or cloth. Call your doctor or clinic or go to an emergency room.

NO ↓

Does he feel something in his eye like dust, dirt, or an eyelash?

YES → Wash your hands. Carefully grab the eyelashes of the upper lid. Now gently pull the upper lid over the lower lid. This will cause tearing, and the foreign particle should be washed out. Repeat if necessary. If the eye is still bothering your child after 10 or 15 minutes, call your doctor or clinic or go to an emergency room.

NO ↓

Was your child hit in the eye?

YES → If the eyeball itself is cut or bleeding, go directly to the emergency room; otherwise put an ice pack or cold cloth over the closed eye. If the eye still hurts, is very red, and is tearing, or if your child has difficulty seeing after one half hour, call your doctor or clinic or go to an emergency room.

NO ↓

If your child is still complaining that his eye is bothering him, call your doctor or clinic or an emergency room.

More about Eye Injuries

The eye is a delicate structure. If you think your child may have suffered a potentially serious eye injury, call your doctor. Do not worry about overreacting. When it comes to the eyes, you really cannot be too careful.

Prevention of Eye Injuries

Eye injury is the most preventable cause of blindness in this country. It is important that your child learn from an early age to wear protective eye gear whenever necessary.

- Make sure your child *always* wears protective eye gear when using any machinery that cuts objects. This includes power saws and drills, chain saws, and lawn mowers.

- Make sure your child *always* wears protective eye gear when playing racquetball or squash.

10. *Fainting*

A person *faints* when he or she collapses suddenly and remains unconscious for a brief period of time.

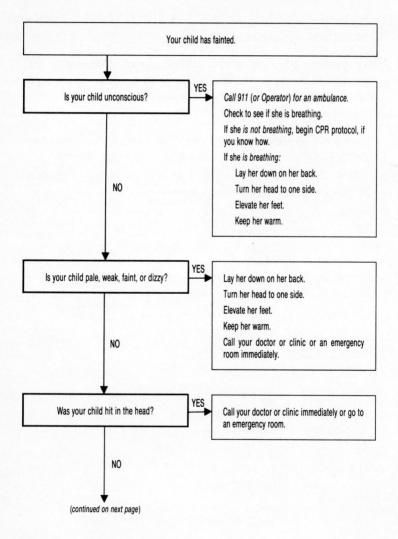

Your child has fainted.

Is your child unconscious? — **YES** →

Call 911 (or Operator) for an ambulance.

Check to see if she is breathing.

If she *is not breathing,* begin CPR protocol, if you know how.

If she *is breathing:*

Lay her down on her back.

Turn her head to one side.

Elevate her feet.

Keep her warm.

NO

Is your child pale, weak, faint, or dizzy? — **YES** →

Lay her down on her back.

Turn her head to one side.

Elevate her feet.

Keep her warm.

Call your doctor or clinic or an emergency room immediately.

NO

Was your child hit in the head? — **YES** →

Call your doctor or clinic immediately or go to an emergency room.

NO

(continued on next page)

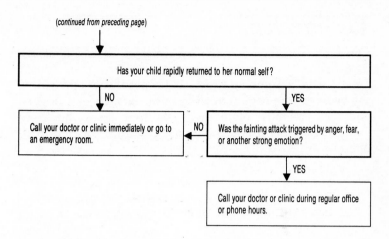

(continued from preceding page)

Has your child rapidly returned to her normal self?

NO

YES

Call your doctor or clinic immediately or go to an emergency room.

NO

Was the fainting attack triggered by anger, fear, or another strong emotion?

YES

Call your doctor or clinic during regular office or phone hours.

More about Fainting

Fainting is caused by a sudden loss of blood flow to the brain. In many instances it is not associated with any medical problem; sometimes it is triggered by a strong emotion such as anger or fear. A teenager who has repeated fainting spells, with no apparent medical problems, may be under significant emotional stress. Fainting can, however, be a symptom of many different illnesses ranging from heart disease to seizures. It is important, therefore, to have a doctor promptly evaluate even a first incident of fainting.

11. *Frostbite*

Frostbite has a numbing effect, so it is not always apparent to the victim at the beginning. The nose, ears, cheeks, fingers, and toes are most often involved; these areas should be checked carefully if you think your child has suffered frostbite.

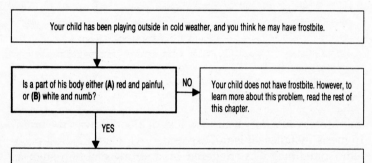

Your child has been playing outside in cold weather, and you think he may have frostbite.

Is a part of his body either **(A)** red and painful, or **(B)** white and numb? **NO** → Your child does not have frostbite. However, to learn more about this problem, read the rest of this chapter.

YES

(A) *If a part of his body is only red and painful, this is a sign that frostbite may develop in a short time.* Follow these directions:

Gently dry the injured area if it is wet.

Rewarm the injured area by blowing on it through cupped hands or by covering it with a warm hand or armpit.

Do not rub the injured area.

Once the injured area is no longer painful, it has been rewarmed. If you have been blowing on the injured area, dry it. If your child is going to stay outside, this part of his body must be recovered with dry clothing.

Take your child indoors if any part of his body should again become red and painful. Rewarm the injured area as above.

or

(B) *Any body parts which are white and numb have frostbite.*

Take your child indoors as soon as possible.

Wrap and keep him as warm and dry as you can until he is brought indoors.

Do not attempt to rewarm any body parts until you are safely indoors and there is no chance that refreezing will happen, because refreezing causes the greatest amount of damage.

(continued on next page)

(continued from preceding page)

↓

Once you are indoors, begin to rewarm the frostbitten areas.

Remove all clothes that are wet or are covering frostbitten areas.

Bathe the area with water that feels warm but not hot to your touch. *Never* use a frostbitten part to test the water temperature. If you have a thermometer, the water should be between 104° and 108° Fahrenheit (40° to 42° Celsius).

Use a large water container so that the frostbitten part does not bump against the sides.

If the area cannot be submerged, apply cloths dipped in warm water and wrung out.

Never use dry-heat sources such as hair dryers or heat lamps for rewarming, because they heat unevenly and are difficult to regulate. *Do not* use a hot-water bottle, since it too will not heat evenly.

Do not rub frostbitten parts.

Do not place your child near a stove or fire, because excessive heat can cause further tissue damage.

Rewarm until the tip of the injured area begins to get back a flushed (red) color. This should take 20 to 30 minutes. The last 10 minutes will be very painful as the frozen nerves begin to work again.

Call your doctor or clinic or an emergency room while you are rewarming the injured part.

Encourage your child to drink warm fluids such as tea or hot chocolate.

Gently dry the injured part. Cover it in warm, soft clothing or towels.

More about Frostbite

Frostbite occurs when body tissues are frozen. This can happen easily when a child is playing out in wet and windy cold weather.

Exposure to cold causes blood vessels to constrict, decreasing the supply of warming blood to the chilled body parts. Without protection the tissues freeze. Young children are at a greater risk for frostbite because they lose body heat very easily. Cold, wet, windy conditions speed up heat loss from the body surface.

Severe frostbite can cause serious, permanent damage. If a deep infection develops, the affected part may have to be amputated.

The parts of the body most susceptible to frostbite are the

small exposed body parts farthest away from large muscles and deep organs (nose, ears, cheeks, fingers, toes). In young children, frostbite may develop on areas of the face under a wet chin strap.

Prevention of Frostbite

- Use several layers of warm clothing. The layers trap air and minimize loss of body heat.

- Keep dry.

- Wear a warm hat. This is very important, because a high percentage of body heat is lost from an uncovered head.

- Good hand and foot protection is also important. Wear glove or mitten liners and two pairs of socks—an extra warm pair over a light pair. Make sure that clothing is not too tight around the wrists and ankles, otherwise the pressure will reduce the flow of vital, warming blood to the hands and feet.

- Watch for the warning signs of frostbite: pain, redness, and tingling. Exposed areas such as the nose and cheeks should be watched carefully.

- Teach family members to check each other for frostbite when outside in winter weather. Because frostbite has a numbing effect, the victim is not always aware of it at the beginning.

12. *Head Injuries*

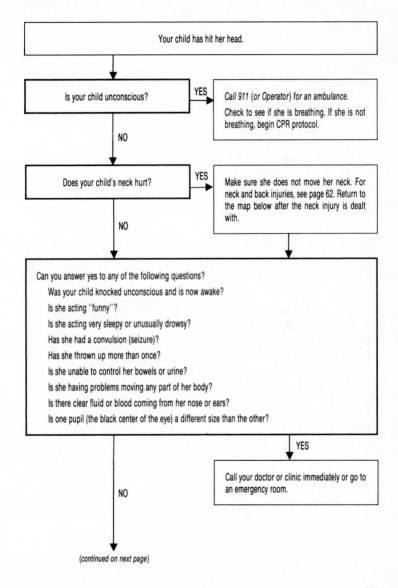

Your child has hit her head.

Is your child unconscious?

YES → *Call 911 (or Operator) for an ambulance.*
Check to see if she is breathing. If she is not breathing, begin CPR protocol.

NO

Does your child's neck hurt?

YES → Make sure she does not move her neck. For neck and back injuries, see page 62. Return to the map below after the neck injury is dealt with.

NO

Can you answer yes to *any* of the following questions?

Was your child knocked unconscious and is now awake?

Is she acting "funny"?

Is she acting very sleepy or unusually drowsy?

Has she had a convulsion (seizure)?

Has she thrown up more than once?

Is she unable to control her bowels or urine?

Is she having problems moving any part of her body?

Is there clear fluid or blood coming from her nose or ears?

Is one pupil (the black center of the eye) a different size than the other?

YES

Call your doctor or clinic immediately or go to an emergency room.

NO

(continued on next page)

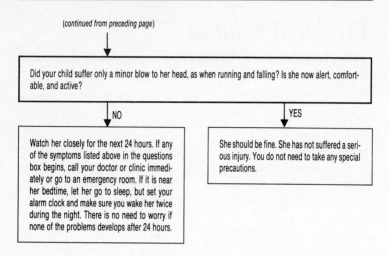

(continued from preceding page)

Did your child suffer only a minor blow to her head, as when running and falling? Is she now alert, comfortable, and active?

NO

Watch her closely for the next 24 hours. If any of the symptoms listed above in the questions box begins, call your doctor or clinic immediately or go to an emergency room. If it is near her bedtime, let her go to sleep, but set your alarm clock and make sure you wake her twice during the night. There is no need to worry if none of the problems develops after 24 hours.

YES

She should be fine. She has not suffered a serious injury. You do not need to take any special precautions.

More about Head Injuries

All children hit their heads at one time or another. Infants learning to walk fall down repeatedly. If your child is walking or running and bangs into something or falls to the ground, this will rarely cause a serious head injury.

It is not unusual for a tender swelling to develop at the injured spot. The swelling may even look alarming, like an egg or golf ball, but it is really not a cause for concern. To help reduce the swelling, apply an ice pack—cracked ice enclosed in a plastic bag, washcloth, or hot-water bottle. Bruises will follow and can last up to a week or more. If your child cuts her scalp, check Chapter 6, "Cuts and Bleeding."

The map at the beginning of this chapter will help you decide if a head injury is serious and will tell you how to handle it.

13. *Heat Illnesses*

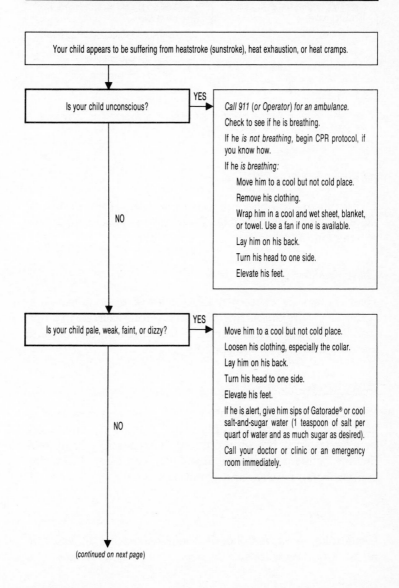

Your child appears to be suffering from heatstroke (sunstroke), heat exhaustion, or heat cramps.

Is your child unconscious?

YES

Call 911 (or Operator) for an ambulance.

Check to see if he is breathing.

If he *is not breathing*, begin CPR protocol, if you know how.

If he *is breathing*:

Move him to a cool but not cold place.

Remove his clothing.

Wrap him in a cool and wet sheet, blanket, or towel. Use a fan if one is available.

Lay him on his back.

Turn his head to one side.

Elevate his feet.

NO

Is your child pale, weak, faint, or dizzy?

YES

Move him to a cool but not cold place.

Loosen his clothing, especially the collar.

Lay him on his back.

Turn his head to one side.

Elevate his feet.

If he is alert, give him sips of Gatorade® or cool salt-and-sugar water (1 teaspoon of salt per quart of water and as much sugar as desired).

Call your doctor or clinic or an emergency room immediately.

NO

(continued on next page)

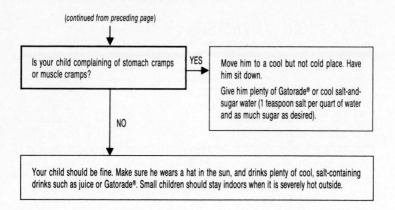

(continued from preceding page)

Is your child complaining of stomach cramps or muscle cramps?

YES → Move him to a cool but not cold place. Have him sit down.

Give him plenty of Gatorade® or cool salt-and-sugar water (1 teaspoon salt per quart of water and as much sugar as desired).

NO

Your child should be fine. Make sure he wears a hat in the sun, and drinks plenty of cool, salt-containing drinks such as juice or Gatorade®. Small children should stay indoors when it is severely hot outside.

More about Heat Illnesses

Overexposure to hot conditions can cause several problems, all of which are preventable. These include heat cramps, heat exhaustion, and heatstroke, or sunstroke.

HEAT CRAMPS

Heat cramps are caused by excessive loss of body salts and water. They are often triggered by vigorous exercise in a hot, dry environment. Heat cramps usually occur in the legs and stomach and can be very painful.

HEAT EXHAUSTION

Heat exhaustion also is caused by excessive loss of body salts and water. It occurs in people who are doing vigorous work or exercise in a hot environment. The possible symptoms include tremendous fatigue, irritability, confusion, headache, stomachache, nausea, and vomiting.

HEATSTROKE

Heatstroke, or sunstroke, is the most severe illness that results from overexposure to heat. It is potentially fatal.

Individuals suffering from heatstroke will get progressively weaker and eventually slip into a coma. Heatstroke is caused by excessive loss of body salts and water accompanied by excessive absorption of environmental heat. It is usually, but not always, associated with vigorous exercise.

As the body temperature rises, more blood is automatically sent to the skin in an attempt to cool the body's central core. In addition, the volume of blood has been reduced by sweating and dehydration. The redistribution of blood to the skin surface, together with sweating and dehydration, acts to reduce the amount of blood available to the heart and brain. When the blood volume drops below a critical level, the brain is affected. This is what causes the coma and creates a potentially fatal situation.

Prevention of Heat Illnesses

- Always wear a hat in strong sunlight.
- Drink plenty of salt-containing fluids during vigorous activity. There is *no* reason to restrict fluids because of fears that drinking will cause cramps. Heat cramps are *caused by* excessive loss of body salts and water.

  Salt-containing fluids include: fruit juices, Gatorade®, and fruit drinks with 1 teaspoon of salt added per quart.
- Only teenagers and adults should use salt tablets. The tablets should *always* be swallowed with plenty of water.
- Keep young children cool indoors when it is severely hot outside.

14. *Neck and Back Injuries*

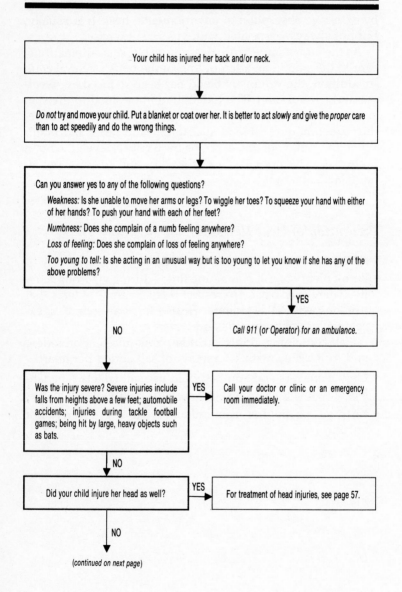

Your child has injured her back and/or neck.

Do not try and move your child. Put a blanket or coat over her. It is better to act *slowly* and give the *proper* care than to act speedily and do the wrong things.

Can you answer yes to *any* of the following questions?

Weakness: Is she unable to move her arms or legs? To wiggle her toes? To squeeze your hand with either of her hands? To push your hand with each of her feet?

Numbness: Does she complain of a numb feeling anywhere?

Loss of feeling: Does she complain of loss of feeling anywhere?

Too young to tell: Is she acting in an unusual way but is too young to let you know if she has any of the above problems?

YES

NO

Call 911 (or Operator) for an ambulance.

Was the injury severe? Severe injuries include falls from heights above a few feet; automobile accidents; injuries during tackle football games; being hit by large, heavy objects such as bats.

YES → Call your doctor or clinic or an emergency room immediately.

NO

Did your child injure her head as well?

YES → For treatment of head injuries, see page 57.

NO

(continued on next page)

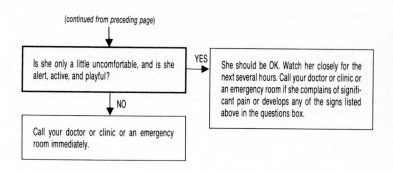

(continued from preceding page)

Is she only a little uncomfortable, and is she alert, active, and playful?

YES → She should be OK. Watch her closely for the next several hours. Call your doctor or clinic or an emergency room if she complains of significant pain or develops any of the signs listed above in the questions box.

NO

Call your doctor or clinic or an emergency room immediately.

More about Neck and Back Injuries

Neck and back injuries have to be examined carefully whenever they occur. If a child is playing and falls to the ground or is punched by another child of the same age, major problems rarely result. However, falls from heights or automobile accidents, even in slow-moving vehicles, can cause real problems.

The spinal cord travels down from the brain through the middle of the spine, or backbone. Nerves in the spinal cord carry signals from the brain to the arms, legs, and all other parts of the body. Normally the bones of the spine form a passage, or canal, that protects the spinal cord and its delicate nerves from injury.

A broken bone in the neck or back causes nerve damage only when the spinal cord is also injured. Some breaks cause injury to the spinal cord only when the broken bone moves. That is why victims of possible neck or back injury *must not be moved* except by trained medical personnel. It is most important not to act quickly without thinking. *Speed is less important than proper care.*

Be very cautious if you think your child has significantly injured her back or neck. If she seems OK but you are not sure, handle the situation as if she *does* have a significant injury. It is much better to feel a little foolish after calling an ambulance for a child who turns out to be OK than to let a child walk away and then develop paralysis or other serious problems later on.

The map at the beginning of the chapter will help you take the proper course of action. It is designed to emphasize caution. This allows you to be confident that you have not missed an important injury and that you have handled the situation correctly.

15. *Poisoning*

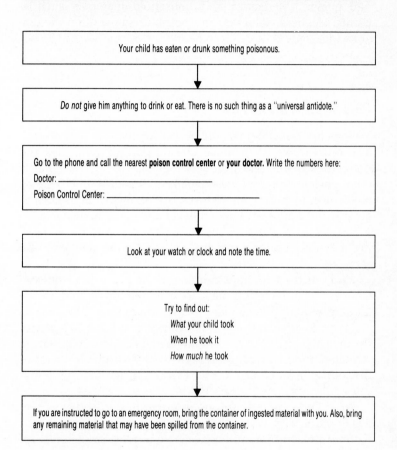

Your child has eaten or drunk something poisonous.

↓

Do not give him anything to drink or eat. There is no such thing as a "universal antidote."

↓

Go to the phone and call the nearest **poison control center** or **your doctor.** Write the numbers here:

Doctor: _____

Poison Control Center: _____

↓

Look at your watch or clock and note the time.

↓

Try to find out:

What your child took

When he took it

How much he took

↓

If you are instructed to go to an emergency room, bring the container of ingested material with you. Also, bring any remaining material that may have been spilled from the container.

More about Poisoning

Poisoning is probably the most common emergency among young children. It occurs most often in children under 5 years of age, especially in children of 1 or 2 years of age. About 2 million American children a year are poisoned by accident, and some of them do die.

Poisoning happens most often in the kitchen, bathroom, and garage. Medicines and household materials such as paints, cleaners, solvents, and polish are most often the poisons ingested.

Poison Prevention Tips

Young children will put *anything and everything in their mouths.* You must make your house safe by putting medicines and dangerous household products high up, *out of reach, out of sight*, enclosed *in child-proof containers.* It is best to lock up all medicines, including all nonprescription medications such as aspirin and nonaspirin pain reliever and fever medicine (acetaminophen). Make sure that there are no dangerous cleaning materials under your sink and that your garage is also safe.

Find out the telephone number of the nearest poison control center and write it next to your telephone and in the space provided on the map for this chapter.

There is no such thing as a "universal antidote." Many of the instructions listed on containers of hazardous material are outdated and incorrect. *Always check* first with your doctor or the local poison control center before giving your child anything following an ingestion.

Buy a bottle of *ipecac* (pronounced: *ip* ah kak) and store it in a safe place with your other medicines. It can be purchased without prescription and is available in most drugstores. Ipecac is a medicine that is used in certain situations to make a person vomit and expel poisonous material from the stomach. It can be dangerous in certain situations, however. So *never* give your child ipecac before speaking to your doctor or the local poison control center.

When your family visits relatives, or when relatives come to visit, especially older family members, be sure to ask if they have any medicines with them. If so, store these medicines safely out of the reach of small children. Remember, pocketbooks often contain medicines. Many accidental poisonings have resulted from a curious toddler eating the "candy" he found in Grandma's purse.

II. *Common Problems and Concerns*

How to Use Medicines

Perhaps you have had this experience, or one similar to it:

You have just been to the doctor with your sick child. As you are about to leave the examining room, the doctor gives you a prescription for her. You don't realize until you're out the door that you're not sure just *exactly* what you are supposed to do. The Latin writing on the prescription is of little help. Of course, the druggist can answer most questions, but directions also should be clearly presented to you by your doctor.

It is very important that you have a clear understanding of the medicines recommended for your child—whether they are over-the-counter medicines such as aspirin, or prescription medicines such as antibiotics. It is also important to tell your doctor if your child has had any allergic reactions to medicines in the past.

These are the items you should have clearly explained by the doctor whenever a medicine is recommended for your child:

WHAT is the medicine supposed to do?

WHERE is it supposed to be given? For example, some ear medicines are placed directly in the ear to relieve ear pain, while some others, such as antibiotics, are given by mouth to fight an ear infection.

HOW OFTEN are you to give the medicine?

WHEN are you to give the medicine? Certain medicines have to be given at exact time intervals, but most medicines allow some flexibility in their timing. Should the medicine be given before meals, after meals, or at any time?

FOR HOW LONG are you supposed to give the medicine?

ARE INTERACTIONS POSSIBLE between this medicine and any other medicines your child may be taking?

Side Effects

Side effects of medicines actually are effects; they just happen to be undesirable effects. Every medicine has side effects. You want to know which ones are expected and acceptable, and which ones are signals that you should stop giving the medicine to your child.

Ask your doctor these questions any time your child is placed on a medicine:

Which side effects are *expected* and *acceptable*?

Which side effects are *signals to stop giving* the medicine?

If you are not sure if your child is experiencing a serious adverse reaction to a medicine, do not give the next dose of medicine. Instead, call your doctor or clinic and find out what you should do.

Tips on Giving Medicine to Children

Almost all medicines can be mixed in a small amount of pleasant-tasting food such as a few teaspoons of applesauce, maple syrup, or ice cream, or an ounce or two of fruit juice. Use whatever works best for you. My older daughter loves ketchup, so we give her medicine mixed in small amounts of ketchup!

Never trick your child by secretly placing medicine in her food.

Do not ask your child if she wants to take her medicine. After all, if she says no, what are you going to do? Why ask her opinion if you are not going to respect her answer? Tell your child it is time for her medicine, or say, "Let's take the medicine."

For an infant or young toddler, you can use an oral syringe or dropper to squirt liquid medicines into the mouth. This method also has the advantage of allowing you to carefully measure the amount of medicine you are giving.

Things to Remember

Keep all medicines high out of children's reach in a locked container.

Never give a child prescription medicines that are left over from a previous illness *unless* instructed to do so by a physician; antibiotics often are misused in this way. It is of no help, and is potentially harmful, to give your child a few doses of an antibiotic every time she gets a cold.

Keep on giving the medicine until you have completed the *full* number of doses prescribed by the doctor. Do not, for example, stop an asthma medicine on the second day of a five-day course because your child is now feeling better.

It is particularly important to give the full number of doses of antibiotics. A child will often feel better several days after an antibiotic has begun to work, but the infection is still present. If the medicine is stopped at this point, your child may well get sick all over again.

How to Use a Thermometer

A thermometer is used to check for fever. A child is feverish when his temperature is above 101° Fahrenheit or 38.3° Celsius, taken orally or rectally. *F* is the abbreviation for Fahrenheit, and *C* is the abbreviation for Celsius.

If your child is ill, and you discover a fever, it is not generally necessary to retake the temperature more often than every four to six hours at most. A child who is alert, active, busy, and playful doesn't need to be checked for fever. To learn more about fever, see Chapter 26, "Fever."

Thermometers are used to take a person's temperature by

mouth (oral temperature), rectum (rectal temperature), or armpit (axillary temperature). Rectal temperature is used mostly for infants, young children, and hospitalized adults. Oral temperatures can be taken once a child is old enough to hold the thermometer in his mouth without biting it, to sit still for at least two minutes, and to keep his mouth closed over the thermometer. Axillary temperatures are not reliable.

Specific, step-by-step instructions are given below for the use of glass, mercury-filled thermometers. Electronic digital thermometers have recently become available. They are expensive, but they are fast and convenient to use.

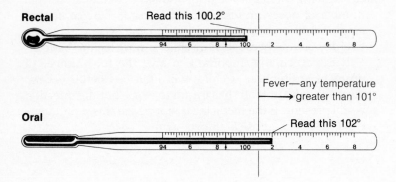

Rectal Read this 100.2°

94 6 8 100 2 4 6 8

Fever—any temperature
→ greater than 101°

Oral Read this 102°

94 6 8 100 2 4 6 8

Preparation:

Shake the thermometer down below 98° Fahrenheit (36.7° Celsius). To do this, hold the thermometer firmly by the top (not the bulb end), and shake it with quick flips of the wrist.

If you are using an oral temperature, make sure your child has had no cold or hot liquids to drink in the past 15 minutes.

To take a temperature by rectum:

Coat bulb end of a rectal thermometer with petroleum jelly. (Rectal thermometers have short, round bulbs.) Spread buttocks so that rectum is easily seen. Gently insert the thermometer at least until the bulb can no longer be seen. *Do not* insert farther than 1 inch. You can grasp the thermometer about 1 inch in from the bulb. This will act as a guard. Hold in place for 2 minutes.

To take a temperature by mouth:

Place the bulb end of an oral thermometer under the tongue a little to one side. (Oral thermometers have long, slim bulbs.) Tell your child to close his lips gently, but not to bite the thermometer. Hold in place for 2 minutes.

Reading the thermometer:

Slowly rotate the thermometer until you can see the line of mercury or alcohol. This will be either silver (mercury) or red or blue (alcohol). Read the thermometer where the line ends.

Cleaning the thermometer:

Never use hot water. Hold the thermometer by the top and clean with warm, soapy water. Wipe down with rubbing alcohol if it is available.

Guidelines for thermometer use:

Always handle the thermometer by the top, not by the bulb end.

Always clean the thermometer after taking someone's temperature.

Never use hot water to clean the thermometer.

Keep the thermometer in its case, out of the reach of children.

What to Do if Your Child Bites on a Thermometer and It Breaks in His Mouth

Occasionally a child will bite on a thermometer, causing it to break. This rarely causes harm, even though the child may have swallowed mercury and some bits of broken glass. The amount of mercury in a thermometer is very small, and only a tiny portion of the swallowed mercury is absorbed into the body; almost all of it leaves the body in bowel movements. So your child cannot possibly be poisoned by a broken mercury thermometer.

Gently rinse out your child's mouth with water and check for any missing pieces of glass. A small amount of bleeding from the gums may occur. This is not dangerous. Your child should be fine. But if you believe your child has swallowed a large piece of glass, or if you have any questions or concerns, call your doctor or clinic.

What to Do if a Rectal Thermometer Breaks while You Are Taking Your Child's Temperature

This is not a dangerous situation. There has never been a report of serious injury caused by a broken rectal thermometer. The mercury, for the reasons mentioned above, poses no risk of poisoning. The broken end of the thermometer is safely encased in feces and will therefore make its way uneventfully out of the body.

How to Choose a Doctor for Your Child

Finding a doctor whom you trust and feel comfortable with can be difficult, whether the doctor is for yourself or for your child. This is a problem parents usually must deal with when expecting their first child or when moving into a new community.

There are three types of doctors qualified to handle the general care of infants, children, and teenagers: pediatricians, family practitioners, and general practitioners. *Pediatricians* are specialists trained in the care of newborns, infants, children, and teenagers. *Family practitioners* are not restricted in their training to younger patients; they deliver babies, do minor surgery, and can care for adults. *General practitioners* are older physicians who were trained in ways somewhat similar to the training of family practitioners. Like family physicians, GPs (as they are called) treat patients of all ages.

Each type of training has its strengths and weaknesses. Pediatricians are the most intensively trained in the care of young people, but they cannot provide care for your entire family. Family practitioners are qualified to give care for the whole family, but they may have difficulty with complicated illnesses in newborns, premature infants, or very young children. General practitioners gain tremendous experience, but they may have difficulty keeping up with the latest techniques.

I have had the privilege of working with outstanding pediatricians, family practitioners, and general practitioners. I've seen that it is not the specific type of training that makes these physicians outstanding, but rather their qualities of judgment, thoroughness, personality, honesty, and availability.

How to Compile a List of Available Doctors

There are many sources you can use, including:

- Friends, neighbors, and relatives
- The school nurse
- The telephone book (the yellow pages list doctors by specialty under the listing "Physicians")
- The newborn (neonate) nursery in your local hospital
- Your county's medical society
- Parents of children in your child's class

What to Consider in Choosing a Doctor

Location.   How long will it take you to get to the doctor's office?

Availability.   When does the doctor have office hours? Does he or she have nighttime and weekend hours? Is there a phone hour, when you can call and speak with the doctor? Who is available in emergency situations, and how do you reach the person?

Group or solo practice.   Some parents may have a strong preference for one over the other. Many group practices are organized to allow your child to see the same doctor each time within certain limitations of scheduling.

Financial considerations.   Inquire about billing procedures and costs for services like routine office visits and shots. You will want to know if your insurance covers the more common charges in the doctor's office. Also, will your insurance payment be accepted as full payment for covered services?

Ways to Decide upon a Specific Doctor or Group

For some parents the decision will be easy. But if you have trouble deciding, narrow the list to the two or three doctors who seem most promising. Then call each doctor's office and speak with the receptionist or nurse, who may be able to answer most of the questions detailed above. If you are still uncertain, ask to speak to the doctor or to one of the members from the group, or make an appointment to meet the doctor. This face-to-face interview should give you a good idea of the qualities of the doctor or group and of how the practice is run.

16. *Bites and Stings*

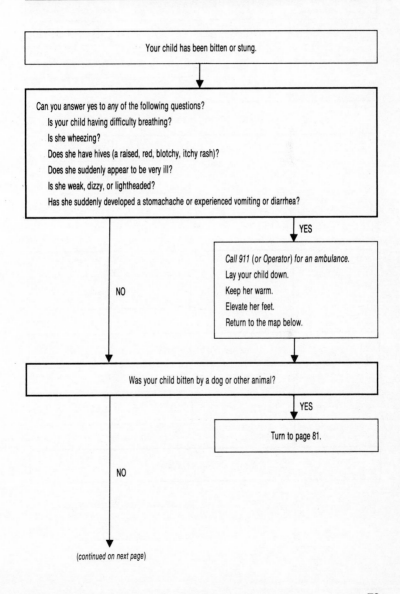

Your child has been bitten or stung.

Can you answer yes to *any* of the following questions?

Is your child having difficulty breathing?

Is she wheezing?

Does she have hives (a raised, red, blotchy, itchy rash)?

Does she suddenly appear to be very ill?

Is she weak, dizzy, or lightheaded?

Has she suddenly developed a stomachache or experienced vomiting or diarrhea?

NO

YES

Call 911 (or Operator) for an ambulance.

Lay your child down.

Keep her warm.

Elevate her feet.

Return to the map below.

Was your child bitten by a dog or other animal?

NO

YES

Turn to page 81.

(continued on next page)

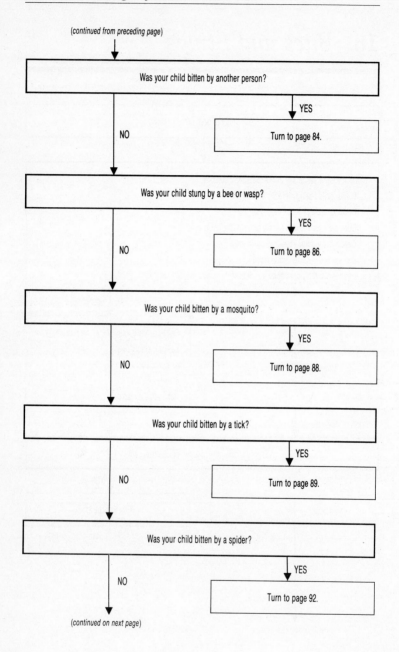

(continued from preceding page)

Was your child bitten by another person?

NO

YES

Turn to page 84.

Was your child stung by a bee or wasp?

NO

YES

Turn to page 86.

Was your child bitten by a mosquito?

NO

YES

Turn to page 88.

Was your child bitten by a tick?

NO

YES

Turn to page 89.

Was your child bitten by a spider?

NO

YES

Turn to page 92.

(continued on next page)

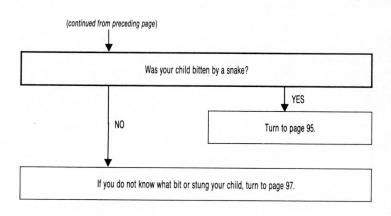

(continued from preceding page)

Was your child bitten by a snake?

NO

YES

Turn to page 95.

If you do not know what bit or stung your child, turn to page 97.

Bites by Dogs and Other Animals

This map deals with bites by dogs and other animals, both pets and wildlife, including foxes, raccoons, coyotes, wolves, bats, skunks, rats, squirrels, mice, gerbils, and hamsters.

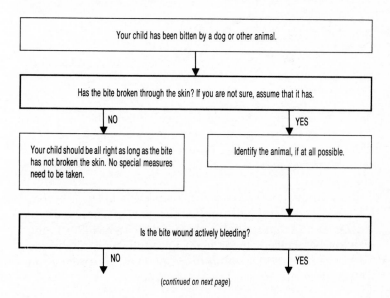

Your child has been bitten by a dog or other animal.

Has the bite broken through the skin? If you are not sure, assume that it has.

NO

Your child should be all right as long as the bite has not broken the skin. No special measures need to be taken.

YES

Identify the animal, if at all possible.

Is the bite wound actively bleeding?

NO

YES

(continued on next page)

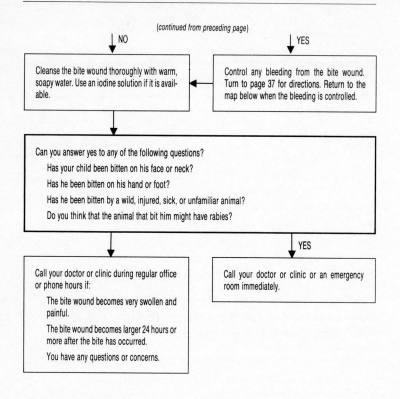

(continued from preceding page)

NO ↓   ↓ **YES**

Cleanse the bite wound thoroughly with warm, soapy water. Use an iodine solution if it is available.

◄── Control any bleeding from the bite wound. Turn to page 37 for directions. Return to the map below when the bleeding is controlled.

Can you answer yes to *any* of the following questions?

Has your child been bitten on his face or neck?

Has he been bitten on his hand or foot?

Has he been bitten by a wild, injured, sick, or unfamiliar animal?

Do you think that the animal that bit him might have rabies?

↓   ↓ **YES**

Call your doctor or clinic during regular office or phone hours if:

The bite wound becomes very swollen and painful.

The bite wound becomes larger 24 hours or more after the bite has occurred.

You have any questions or concerns.

Call your doctor or clinic or an emergency room immediately.

More about Bites by Dogs and Other Animals

Bites by dogs and other animals pose two problems: (1) the injury from the wound itself and (2) the possibility of infection. Animal bites are often preventable. See the end of this section for measures you can take to prevent your child from being bitten.

Bites on the hands and feet are especially likely to become infected. Treatment with antibiotics may be necessary for large bites. A tetanus shot is given if the bitten child's immunization has lapsed. If the child (or adult) was fully immunized against tetanus within the last 10 years, he is still protected.

RABIES

Rabies is caused by an infection with a type of germ called a *virus*. In humans rabies is almost always the result of a bite by an animal that is itself infected with the rabies virus. Untreated rabies is almost always fatal. Children are more likely than adults to get rabies. They tend to approach animals, and their small size makes them less able to defend themselves from animal bites.

In the United States, rabies most commonly results from bites by skunks, bats, raccoons, and foxes. Dogs and cats rarely carry the virus. And, contrary to popular belief, rodents such as rats, squirrels, and mice also rarely carry rabies. Fortunately, incidences of the disease are very uncommon in the United States.

It is not always possible to tell from an animal's behavior whether or not it has rabies. Rabid animals do not always foam at the mouth and act irritably. Indeed, wild animals infected with rabies may be overly friendly. The only way to confirm rabies in an animal is to catch the animal and subject it to special medical tests.

When rabies is proved or strongly suspected, the bite victim is given a vaccine. This form of treatment is possible because it takes a very long time after the bite for the symptoms of rabies to appear. The vaccine works by building up the body's infection-fighting defenses. It is given in multiple shots in the arm or thigh (not in the abdomen) over a period of a couple of weeks. The latest rabies vaccine causes a minimal degree of discomfort and rarely causes serious side effects. Pain, swelling, and tenderness may occur around the shot area for a few days. Fever and upset stomach may occur for a couple days after each shot. All of these problems are minor and temporary.

It is not always possible to catch and test a wild animal that has bitten a child. However, if rabies is strongly suspected, as in a skunk or bat bite, the vaccine should be given.

At times the decision to treat a child for rabies is difficult to make. Each situation should be evaluated carefully by the doctor, with input from the parents of the child, the child himself (if he is old enough), and expert doctors who specialize in treating childhood infections.

Prevention of Animal Bites

- Avoid all unfamiliar, wild, sick, or injured animals.
- Do not take in stray animals.
- Have your own pets vaccinated.
- Report any unfamiliar, wild, sick, or injured animal to the police.
- Do not let children break up an animal fight even if it involves your own pet. An adult should use a rake, broom, or other object to separate the animals.

Human Bites

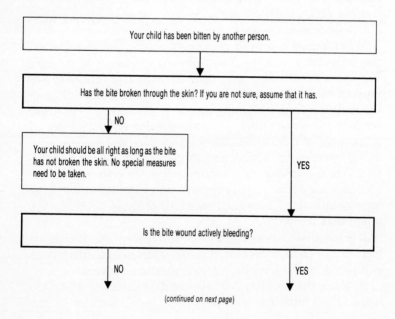

Your child has been bitten by another person.

Has the bite broken through the skin? If you are not sure, assume that it has.

NO

Your child should be all right as long as the bite has not broken the skin. No special measures need to be taken.

YES

Is the bite wound actively bleeding?

NO   **YES**

(continued on next page)

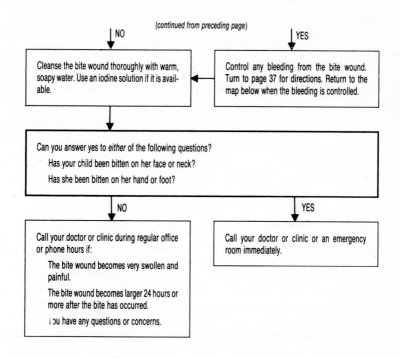

(continued from preceding page)

NO | **YES**

Cleanse the bite wound thoroughly with warm, soapy water. Use an iodine solution if it is available.

Control any bleeding from the bite wound. Turn to page 37 for directions. Return to the map below when the bleeding is controlled.

Can you answer yes to *either* of the following questions?

   Has your child been bitten on her face or neck?

   Has she been bitten on her hand or foot?

NO | **YES**

Call your doctor or clinic during regular office or phone hours if:

   The bite wound becomes very swollen and painful.

   The bite wound becomes larger 24 hours or more after the bite has occurred.

   You have any questions or concerns.

Call your doctor or clinic or an emergency room immediately.

More about Human Bites

Human bites are often more dangerous than animal bites as a cause of injury and infection. It may be necessary to give an antibiotic by mouth for a brief period following a bite by another person. A tetanus shot is indicated if the bitten child is overdue for her immunization.

The hand is the part of the body most frequently bitten in human contact; usually the bite results from a fist hitting an opponent's teeth. Cleaning the wound is very important. For deep bites this may require an injection of local anesthesia. Stitches are rarely used, because they close in the infection.

Bee and Wasp Stings

This section deals with stings by honeybees, wasps, yellow jackets, and hornets.

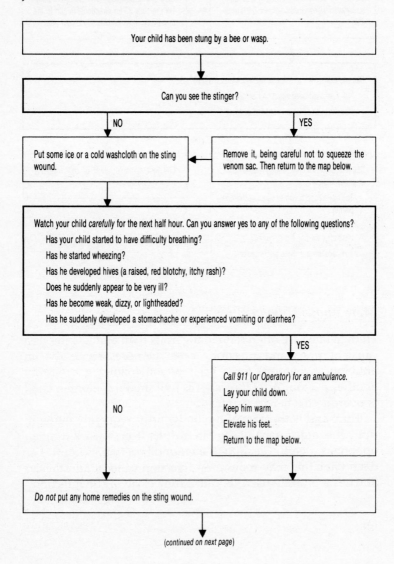

Your child has been stung by a bee or wasp.

Can you see the stinger?

NO

Put some ice or a cold washcloth on the sting wound.

YES

Remove it, being careful not to squeeze the venom sac. Then return to the map below.

Watch your child *carefully* for the next half hour. Can you answer yes to *any* of the following questions?

Has your child started to have difficulty breathing?

Has he started wheezing?

Has he developed hives (a raised, red blotchy, itchy rash)?

Does he suddenly appear to be very ill?

Has he become weak, dizzy, or lightheaded?

Has he suddenly developed a stomachache or experienced vomiting or diarrhea?

YES

Call 911 (or Operator) for an ambulance.

Lay your child down.

Keep him warm.

Elevate his feet.

Return to the map below.

NO

Do not put any home remedies on the sting wound.

(continued on next page)

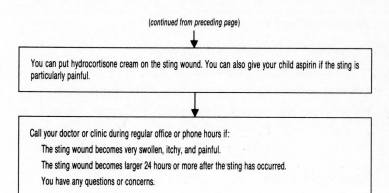

(continued from preceding page)

You can put hydrocortisone cream on the sting wound. You can also give your child aspirin if the sting is particularly painful.

Call your doctor or clinic during regular office or phone hours if:

The sting wound becomes very swollen, itchy, and painful.

The sting wound becomes larger 24 hours or more after the sting has occurred.

You have any questions or concerns.

More about Bee and Wasp Stings

Bee and wasp stings can be very painful, but in most cases they are not dangerous. Most stings can be handled with a few simple measures at home.

Rarely, however, a child or adult will develop a severe allergic reaction to a sting. The most troublesome insects belong to the Hymenoptera (pronounced: high muh *nop* tuh ruh) group, which includes honeybees, wasps, yellow jackets, hornets, and fire ants.

The symptoms of a severe allergic reaction are listed on the preceding map. This type of reaction always develops within the first half hour after a sting. The medical terms for this type of severe allergic reaction are *anaphylaxis* (pronounced anna fuh *lack* suss) and *anaphylactic* (pronounced: anna fuh *lack* tic) *shock*.

Any child with a history of a severe allergic reaction to a sting should receive a careful medical evaluation. He should carry a specially prepared, preloaded syringe containing epinephrine (adrenaline). The child and his parents should be instructed in its proper use. It may be necessary to give the child a series of allergy shots to protect him from a future severe allergic reaction.

Prevention of Bee and Wasp Stings

- Don't wear bright-colored clothing.
- Don't walk around with bare feet.
- Avoid wearing short-sleeved shirts and shorts.
- Don't use hair sprays, deodorants, perfumes, cologne, or scented soaps, which attract insects.

Mosquito Bites

Mosquito bites can be a terrible nuisance and cause great discomfort, especially in young children. Thanks to disease-control measures in the United States, mosquito bites are almost never dangerous.

Treatment of Mosquito Bites

1. Give your child a cool bath.
2. Paint the bites with calamine or an equivalent brand of lotion, or put hydrocortisone cream on the bites. These medicines can be purchased without a prescription. Call your doctor or clinic if the itching becomes particularly severe. The doctor may prescribe an oral antihistamine preparation such as Benadryl® or Atarax®. Be aware, however, that antihistamines can cause drowsiness and excessive sleeping.
3. Cut your child's fingernails short so the bites can't be scratched open.

Prevention of Mosquito Bites

- Wear a long-sleeved shirt with the collar buttoned or one that has a turtleneck.
- Avoid hair sprays, deodorants, perfumes, colognes, and scented soaps, which attract insects.
- Use an insect repellent.

Tick Bites

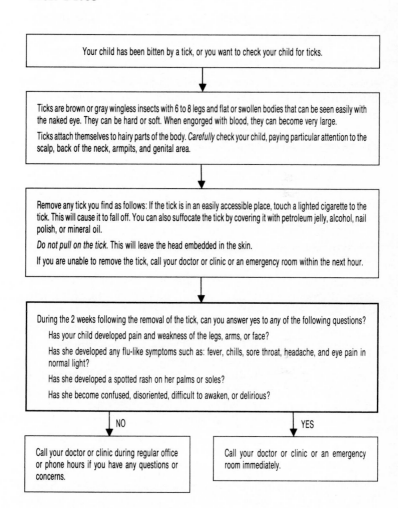

Your child has been bitten by a tick, or you want to check your child for ticks.

Ticks are brown or gray wingless insects with 6 to 8 legs and flat or swollen bodies that can be seen easily with the naked eye. They can be hard or soft. When engorged with blood, they can become very large.

Ticks attach themselves to hairy parts of the body. *Carefully* check your child, paying particular attention to the scalp, back of the neck, armpits, and genital area.

Remove any tick you find as follows: If the tick is in an easily accessible place, touch a lighted cigarette to the tick. This will cause it to fall off. You can also suffocate the tick by covering it with petroleum jelly, alcohol, nail polish, or mineral oil.

Do not pull on the tick. This will leave the head embedded in the skin.

If you are unable to remove the tick, call your doctor or clinic or an emergency room within the next hour.

During the 2 weeks following the removal of the tick, can you answer yes to *any* of the following questions?

Has your child developed pain and weakness of the legs, arms, or face?

Has she developed any flu-like symptoms such as: fever, chills, sore throat, headache, and eye pain in normal light?

Has she developed a spotted rash on her palms or soles?

Has she become confused, disoriented, difficult to awaken, or delirious?

NO

Call your doctor or clinic during regular office or phone hours if you have any questions or concerns.

YES

Call your doctor or clinic or an emergency room immediately.

More about Tick Bites

Ticks are bloodsucking insects that can pass infections on to humans. The bite from a tick may not be very painful. The danger is from the infection that may follow a tick bite.

Ticks are found in large numbers in the forests of the east coast from Massachusetts to Florida, in the southeast, and in the midwest. They are concentrated most heavily in and around Maryland.

Tick fever and tick paralysis are the types of infections that can result from a tick bite. The infection usually occurs within a week of the bite.

TICK FEVER

The symptoms of tick fever include flu-like symptoms, which may be accompanied by stomachaches, muscle aches, joint pains, and nosebleeds. Headache and eye pain in normal light are usually prominent. A spotted rash on the palms and soles may occur as well.

Tick fever can be treated effectively during hospitalization with antibiotics given through the veins. A vaccine is available for individuals who are at high risk.

Rocky Mountain spotted fever is one type of tick fever. The name is poorly chosen, since the fever most commonly occurs on the east coast and rarely occurs in the Rockies.

TICK PARALYSIS

This condition is marked by progressive paralysis; usually, the area first affected is the legs, followed by the arms, breathing muscles, and face. The suspected cause of the disease is a chemical toxin released by female ticks. Paralysis occurs typically one to five days after a tick bite and can progress very rapidly. Removal of the tick early in the course of the disease is followed by prompt improvement.

LYME DISEASE

Lyme disease or Lyme arthritis is a form of arthritis that can occur in children. The disease was first described in Lyme, Connecticut about 10 years ago. The disease commonly occurs in the northeast, particularly southern New England and Long Island.

The disease is spread by a type of small tick. Three days to three weeks following the tick bite, a characteristic rash develops at the site of the bite. The rash turns into a large expanding red patch that is either flat or raised. It may become very large, up to 8 inches or more in diameter. The edges of the rash may be redder than the center. The rash may burn, but is usually not itchy or very painful. Headache, fever, chills, and lack of energy may accompany the rash.

Several weeks following the rash, arthritis often develops. A few large joints, especially the knees, become red, hot, swollen and painful. The arthritis lasts several days, and may disappear and return several weeks later. The arthritis can persist, although rarely, for several years.

Another rare complication of Lyme disease is meningitis or meningoencephalitis (meningitis with confusion and disorientation). This usually occurs days to weeks after the rash. Lack of balance and other problems may occur at the same time. The symptoms last several weeks and may recur.

Antibiotics, given when the rash occurs, may shorten the duration of the rash and prevent or reduce the chances of subsequent arthritis or neurologic complications. All but a few individuals eventually recover completely, even after repeated attacks of arthritis or neurologic complications.

Prevention of Tick Bites

Ticks are most commonly picked up in the woods or from tick-infested dogs. The following preventive measures are called for in areas where ticks are found in great numbers:

• Wear a hat and keep the back of your neck covered when in the woods.

• Check your children and yourself carefully after being in the woods. Pay special attention to the back of the neck.

• Dogs should wear tick collars. A dog's tick collar should be replaced every one to two months.

• Dogs should be checked daily for ticks to prevent an infestation of the home. If ticks are found, they should be removed as described on the map.

• Outdoor clothing can be impregnated with tick repellent.

Spider Bites

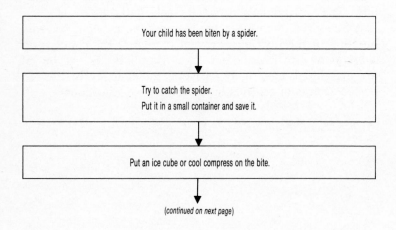

Your child has been bitten by a spider.

Try to catch the spider.
Put it in a small container and save it.

Put an ice cube or cool compress on the bite.

(continued on next page)

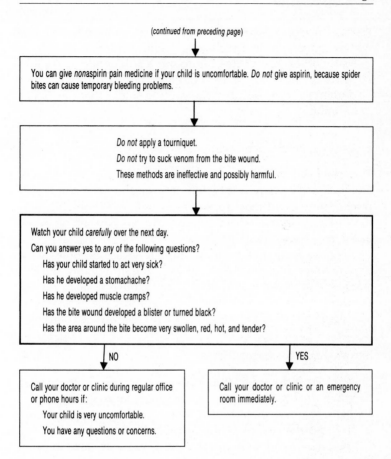

(continued from preceding page)

You can give *nonaspirin* pain medicine if your child is uncomfortable. *Do not* give aspirin, because spider bites can cause temporary bleeding problems.

Do not apply a tourniquet.

Do not try to suck venom from the bite wound.

These methods are ineffective and possibly harmful.

Watch your child *carefully* over the next day.

Can you answer yes to *any* of the following questions?

Has your child started to act very sick?

Has he developed a stomachache?

Has he developed muscle cramps?

Has the bite wound developed a blister or turned black?

Has the area around the bite become very swollen, red, hot, and tender?

NO

Call your doctor or clinic during regular office or phone hours if:

Your child is very uncomfortable.

You have any questions or concerns.

YES

Call your doctor or clinic or an emergency room immediately.

More about Spider Bites

Most spider bites can be managed easily and safely at home without any special measures.

Contrary to popular belief, most spiders are harmless; they prefer to avoid human contact. When a spider bite causes a problem, it is due to a chemical toxin the spider released into the bite wound. In the continental United States there are two types of poisonous spiders commonly encountered: the black widow and the brown recluse, or violin spider.

Many other insect bites can mimic a spider bite, including bites from sand flies, fleas, bedbugs, ticks, and mites. It is important to try to identify the specific spider that has bitten your child.

BLACK WIDOW SPIDER BITES

The black widow spider is found throughout the United States. The bite may not be felt; it is said to resemble a pinprick. The wound may appear as a slight swelling with two tiny red dots in the center. Intense pain and throbbing occur in the area soon after the bite.

Over the next several hours the bite victim becomes very sick with severe stomach cramps, vomiting, and muscle cramps. Convulsions and loss of consciousness may result. Hospitalization is required so that vigorous, supportive care may be given. Death rarely results, and recovery is complete.

BROWN RECLUSE SPIDER BITES

This spider is found in the midwest and the south central region of the United States. Its bite causes little or no immediate pain, but over the next few hours symptoms appear similar to those that follow a bite by a black widow.

The bite wound soon develops a blister with surrounding blanched (pale white) and red rings, somewhat like a bull's-eye target. The center of the wound may develop a large black crusty scab, which in turn becomes an ulcer. This ulcer may take several weeks to heal and can leave a significant scar.

Brown recluse spider bites can require hospitalization. Fatalities are rare, and recovery is complete.

Snakebites

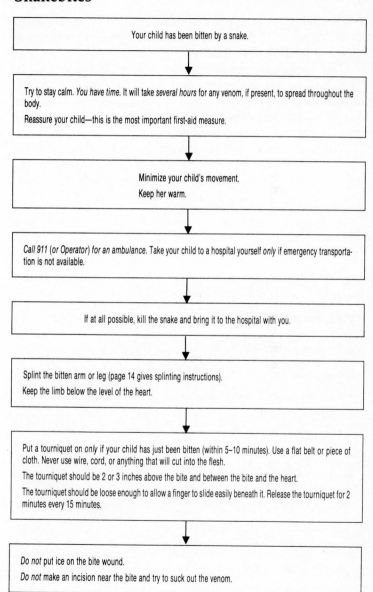

Your child has been bitten by a snake.

Try to stay calm. *You have time.* It will take *several hours* for any venom, if present, to spread throughout the body.

Reassure your child—this is the most important first-aid measure.

Minimize your child's movement.

Keep her warm.

Call 911 (or Operator) for an ambulance. Take your child to a hospital yourself *only* if emergency transportation is not available.

If at all possible, kill the snake and bring it to the hospital with you.

Splint the bitten arm or leg (page 14 gives splinting instructions).

Keep the limb below the level of the heart.

Put a tourniquet on *only* if your child has just been bitten (within 5–10 minutes). Use a flat belt or piece of cloth. Never use wire, cord, or anything that will cut into the flesh.

The tourniquet should be 2 or 3 inches above the bite and between the bite and the heart.

The tourniquet should be loose enough to allow a finger to slide easily beneath it. Release the tourniquet for 2 minutes every 15 minutes.

Do not put ice on the bite wound.

Do not make an incision near the bite and try to suck out the venom.

More about Snakebites

While snakebites are potentially fatal, the survival rate in the United States is high. Children and teenage boys are the most common victims of snakebites.

Most snakes are not poisonous. Almost all the venomous bites in this country are caused by three types of snakes: rattlesnakes, copperheads, and water moccasins, which all belong to the class called *pit vipers*. Rarely does a coral snake or an exotic pet snake bite someone.

Snakebites are almost always on the arms or legs. Poisonous bites occur most commonly and are most severe during the early spring. The southeastern United States is the area where venomous bites are most frequently reported.

Prevention of Snakebites

Children and adults should observe the following points when in a snake-infested area:

- Wear boots and long trousers.
- Never walk barefooted.
- Do not play or explore under ledges or in holes where a snake may hide.

Unidentified Bites

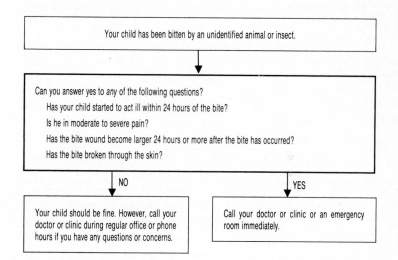

Your child has been bitten by an unidentified animal or insect.

Can you answer yes to *any* of the following questions?

Has your child started to act ill within 24 hours of the bite?

Is he in moderate to severe pain?

Has the bite wound become larger 24 hours or more after the bite has occurred?

Has the bite broken through the skin?

NO

Your child should be fine. However, call your doctor or clinic during regular office or phone hours if you have any questions or concerns.

YES

Call your doctor or clinic or an emergency room immediately.

17. *Car Sickness*

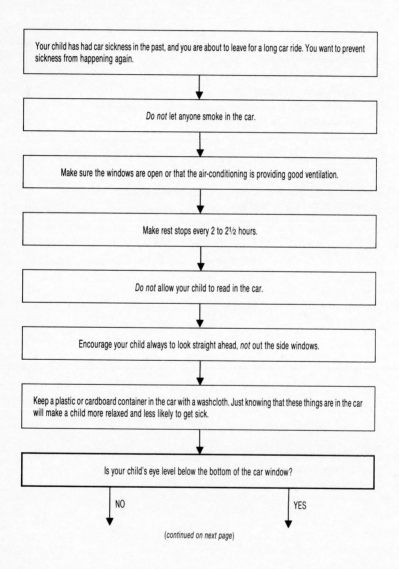

Your child has had car sickness in the past, and you are about to leave for a long car ride. You want to prevent sickness from happening again.

↓

Do not let anyone smoke in the car.

↓

Make sure the windows are open or that the air-conditioning is providing good ventilation.

↓

Make rest stops every 2 to 2½ hours.

↓

Do not allow your child to read in the car.

↓

Encourage your child always to look straight ahead, *not* out the side windows.

↓

Keep a plastic or cardboard container in the car with a washcloth. Just knowing that these things are in the car will make a child more relaxed and less likely to get sick.

↓

Is your child's eye level below the bottom of the car window?

NO   YES

(continued on next page)

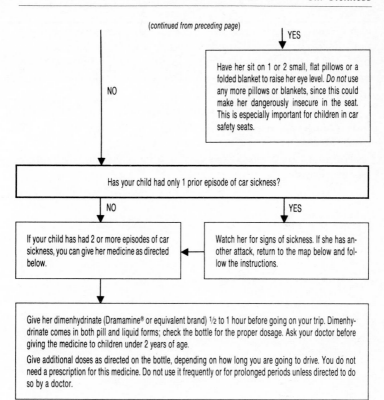

(continued from preceding page)

YES

NO

Have her sit on 1 or 2 small, flat pillows or a folded blanket to raise her eye level. *Do not* use any more pillows or blankets, since this could make her dangerously insecure in the seat. This is especially important for children in car safety seats.

Has your child had only 1 prior episode of car sickness?

NO

YES

If your child has had 2 or more episodes of car sickness, you can give her medicine as directed below.

Watch her for signs of sickness. If she has another attack, return to the map below and follow the instructions.

Give her dimenhydrinate (Dramamine® or equivalent brand) ½ to 1 hour before going on your trip. Dimenhydrinate comes in both pill and liquid forms; check the bottle for the proper dosage. Ask your doctor before giving the medicine to children under 2 years of age.

Give additional doses as directed on the bottle, depending on how long you are going to drive. You do not need a prescription for this medicine. Do not use it frequently or for prolonged periods unless directed to do so by a doctor.

More about Car Sickness

Car sickness, seasickness, and airsickness are all different types of motion sickness. The cause of motion sickness is not known. It is clear, however, that for some reason the balance system in the inner ear is more sensitive to movement in some people than in others.

Children are more likely to become carsick, and adults are more likely to become seasick or airsick. Children usually outgrow car sickness by the time they are teenagers.

Certain things make car sickness worse or more likely to happen. These include cigarette smoke, poor ventilation, quick changes in speed or direction, anxiety, reading, long periods of driving without a break, and bouncing up and down. The effect of bouncing is increased when one can barely see out the window and the landscape keeps coming in and out of view.

It is fine to let your child eat before going on a long car ride, but avoid large meals where a child may overeat and get an upset stomach.

The map for car sickness can also be used for seasickness or airsickness.

18. *Child Abuse*

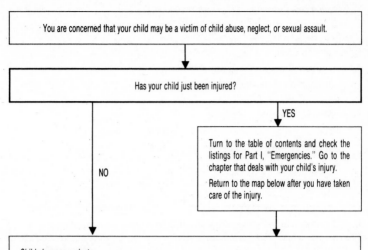

You are concerned that your child may be a victim of child abuse, neglect, or sexual assault.

Has your child just been injured?

YES

Turn to the table of contents and check the listings for Part I, "Emergencies." Go to the chapter that deals with your child's injury.

Return to the map below after you have taken care of the injury.

NO

Child abuse or neglect:

A child under 18 years of age has suffered child abuse or neglect if he has not been given reasonable care and protection. Specific examples include:

Intentionally causing physical injury.

Creating a substantial risk of physical injury.

Failing to give a child adequate food, shelter, clothing, education, or medical care *when able* to do so either through personal resources or public assistance.

Depriving a child of adequate emotional support by continual rejection, scapegoating, or terrorization.

Leaving an infant or child unattended for long periods of time.

Sexual assault:

Sexual assault of a child is the forcing of sexual contact.

In children, sexual contact may involve handling of the child's genitals (penis or vagina) or requests for handling made by an older child or adult. The contact may be oral sex. Sometimes there is an attempt to penetrate the vagina or anus, and penetration may actually occur.

A child may be forced to look at the genitals of an older child or adult, or the child may be asked or told to undress or otherwise expose himself, or to pose for pornographic photos.

(continued on next page)

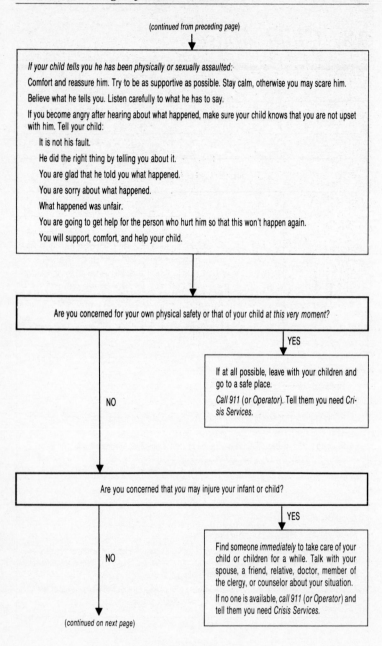

(continued from preceding page)

If your child tells you he has been physically or sexually assaulted:

Comfort and reassure him. Try to be as supportive as possible. Stay calm, otherwise you may scare him.

Believe what he tells you. Listen carefully to what he has to say.

If you become angry after hearing about what happened, make sure your child knows that you are not upset with him. Tell your child:

It is not his fault.

He did the right thing by telling you about it.

You are glad that he told you what happened.

You are sorry about what happened.

What happened was unfair.

You are going to get help for the person who hurt him so that this won't happen again.

You will support, comfort, and help your child.

Are you concerned for your own physical safety or that of your child *at this very moment?*

YES

If at all possible, leave with your children and go to a safe place.

Call 911 (or Operator). Tell them you need *Crisis Services.*

NO

Are you concerned that *you* may injure your infant or child?

YES

Find someone *immediately* to take care of your child or children for a while. Talk with your spouse, a friend, relative, doctor, member of the clergy, or counselor about your situation.

If no one is available, *call 911 (or Operator)* and tell them you need *Crisis Services.*

NO

(continued on next page)

(continued from preceding page)

Having your child examined by a doctor:

If your child has been physically injured, if the vagina or anus has been penetrated, or if clear marks of injury are present, your child should be examined by a doctor. Evidence such as photographs will be taken as part of the examination.

Medical professionals by law *must* report any case of *suspected* child abuse or neglect. A child protection service then becomes involved.

By going to the doctor, you are relieved of the duty of making a report. The doctor makes the report. Your child does not have to show any signs of physical injury for this method of reporting to be used.

You may want to go to your family doctor or pediatrician. If you are not comfortable with these options, you can use an emergency room.

More about reporting:

This can be a very difficult decision because the offender is probably well known to you and your child. You may want to consider the following:

The situation probably did not develop suddenly, out of the blue. More likely, it developed gradually, and the incident will probably be repeated over and over again if nothing is done.

Child abuse and sexual assault are serious crimes, no matter how young the child is or who the offender is.

You may be concerned that your child is too young to give a detailed story that will be believed by the authorities.

You may also be concerned that your child will be subjected to further severe emotional trauma by the reporting process.

The legal system has concern for your child. He will be believed. He will not be asked to repeat indiscriminately what happened. The officials involved will have some understanding and training in working with children.

Who you can call to help you make a report:

A friend or relative.

A hot line or center for people in crisis or victims of domestic violence, child abuse, or rape.

Your doctor or clinic or an emergency room.

Government services for child protection or child welfare.

The police department.

Your minister, rabbi, or priest.

It is fine to talk with others about reporting, but don't let anyone talk you out of reporting if that is what you have decided to do. If you feel that something is wrong, make a report.

(continued on next page)

(continued from preceding page)

Look on the inside cover of your phone book for the toll-free number for reporting child abuse and maltreatment. You can also dial *800-555-1212* to find out the number of a local hot line, or *dial 911 (or Operator)* and ask for *Crisis Services.*

When you make a report, let the officials know at the beginning if you wish to make your report anonymously.

Read the rest of the chapter to learn more about child abuse and sexual assault and what you can do to prevent them.

More about Child Abuse

Child abuse and neglect are serious, wide-spread problems. Almost 1 million cases of child abuse and neglect are reported each year in this country. There are many more cases annually that go unreported.

Neglect of children is the biggest problem. Neglect includes the failure to provide adequate food, shelter, clothing, medical care, supervision to ensure safety, and—most important of all—the failure to provide adequate emotional and psychological support. Emotional deprivation and psychological abuse cause more people to suffer lifelong emotional and mental handicaps than does any other form of maltreatment.

Most abused or neglected children are under 4 years of age, but many are in the 10- to 18-year-old age group. Boys and girls are equally affected. The victimized child is often very different from the other children in the family. A chronically ill, crippled, or retarded child or a premature infant is at a much greater risk of being abused. It is very rare for every child in a family to be victimized by child abuse.

Parents who abuse their children were often victims themselves during their childhood years. In the view of some researchers, these people abuse their children as a way of "working through" their own childhood trauma by repeating the experience, with the difference that they are now in control of the situation.

Offending parents are more likely to be socially isolated and under financial stress. Abusive parents generally love their children but are unable to manage them. They may also have difficulty managing their own lives—such things as a home, job, finances, and relationships with other adults. It doesn't follow, however, that child abuse is a problem solely of the financially disadvantaged. Anyone can be an abuser, even rich, socially active, socially successful individuals.

Sexual Abuse

The problem of the sexual abuse of children has only recently gained national attention. It is an area that had been taboo and is still taboo in many ways.

There are many myths about childhood sexual abuse. It is wrongly supposed that the greatest threat is from a "stranger luring little girls with candy." Experts estimate that 9 out of 10 times the offender is *well known* to the child and family. Offenders are usually friends, relatives, or acquaintances. A teenage girl may be the victim of her date. While girls are more frequently the objects of sexual abuse, the problem exists for children of both sexes.

Sexual abuse is rarely a single isolated incident in a young person's life. It usually develops gradually over an extended period of time and happens over and over again, often for many years.

In my professional experience I have worked with several children and young adults who were victims of childhood sexual abuse. I am glad to say that the climate for identifying and treating child abuse has improved and is still changing for the better. Awareness among health care professionals, teachers, social workers, and adults from all walks of life is increasing.

Prevention of Child Abuse and Neglect

It is most important to offer assistance and support to a family that shows a high level of stress or other problems. The most effective assistance is given in a nonaccusatory manner. Available community services may include family counseling, parenting classes, discipline counseling, crisis intervention, and day-care facilities. Usually it is the reporting of a suspected case of child abuse or neglect that first brings a family into contact with these community services. For this reason, continued emphasis on the reporting of suspected cases of child abuse and neglect remains a cornerstone of prevention.

WHAT TO LOOK FOR

Children may hint at physical, psychological, or sexual abuse in subtle ways. The following signals may indicate that your child is troubled or worried (though, of course, the problem may be something other than abuse):

Having problems with sleeping

Having trouble eating and experiencing a loss of appetite.

Suffering from frequent stomachaches.

Strongly resisting going to a certain baby-sitter's house, or becoming very upset on learning that the sitter is coming over.

Not wanting to go to a particular friend's or relative's house.

Suddenly developing all kinds of new fears.

Suddenly returning to younger, babylike patterns of behavior.

Children may tell you in their own way. A child may simply say, "I don't like Mr. Green anymore." Sometimes the statement will seem vague or strange, as when a child says, for example, "Mr. Thomas has special underwear."

WHAT YOU CAN DO TO PROTECT YOUR CHILD FROM SEXUAL ABUSE

Children *can be taught* to protect themselves from sexual abuse. It is a subject that can be properly discussed beginning at the elementary school level. If children know what to expect, they will be less vulnerable.

Perhaps you are hesitant to talk with your child about this subject. Remember that accurate information given in a sensitive, nonthreatening manner is much less frightening than the ideas children already may have gained from their own imaginations, peers, television, and the movies.

TIPS FOR TALKING TO CHILDREN ABOUT SEXUAL ABUSE

Be specific. Simply telling your child, "Don't take candy from strangers" or, "Don't accept rides from strangers," is not enough. First of all, your child will want to know *why*. Besides, it is not usually a stranger but someone the child knows who tricks, fools, or scares him into performing a sexual act. Use whatever terms you are comfortable with: *penis, vagina, private parts, genitals, between your legs, breasts,* etc. Point to what you mean so the child gets a clear idea.

No secrets. Let your child know that you are always willing and glad to listen to him, that no one should ask him to keep a secret from you. If he is ever worried, upset, scared, confused, or if he gets that "uh-oh" feeling about someone, he should tell you.

Talk about touch. Talk to your child about being touched in ways that are good, ways that are confusing, and ways that are bad.

Some examples of *good touch:*

A hug from Grandma

A goodnight kiss from Mom or Dad

A gentle handshake

A pat on the back

Some examples of *confusing touch:*

A handshake that lasts too long

"Accidental" brushing up against a girl's breasts

A pat on the bottom

A hug that feels too close

Some examples of *bad touch:*

A hard slap on the back

Tickling that does not stop

Grabbing or squeezing breasts

A hand placed in the crotch or between the legs

Having someone place a young person's hand in his or her crotch

Grabbing or squeezing someone's bottom

A hug from behind where the offender presses his or her crotch up against the young person's bottom

How to say "stop." Talk about personal safety. Explain that your child can take care of himself by telling you if a bad or confusing touch happens. Let him know, in terms that he can understand, that he has rights. Here are a few examples of advice you can give your child:

If someone touches you in a way that makes you uncomfortable, you can tell them to stop.

If a person pretends to touch you by accident, it's OK to let them know you don't like it and you want it to stop.

You can firmly lift someone's hand off your body if you feel uncomfortable.

It is very difficult for any parent to discuss this topic, even when an excellent relationship exists between child and parent. You may want to practice first before a mirror, or with your spouse, or even with one of your child's stuffed animals.

You may want to read more about ways to talk with your children about sexual abuse before bringing up the subject. Two excellent sources are the short pamphlets, *He Told Me Not to Tell* ($2.50) and *Touch and Sexual Abuse* (20 cents). These and other helpful pamphlets can be obtained from Network Publications, 1700 Mission Street, Suite 204, P.O. Box 8506, Santa Cruz, CA 95061-8506. (Send 15 percent extra for shipping and handling.)

19. *Colds*

Symptoms of the common cold include runny nose, sinus congestion, fever, mild sore throat, sneezing, cough, and headache.

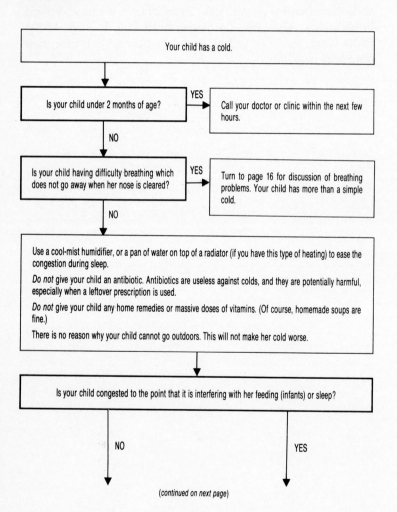

Your child has a cold.

Is your child under 2 months of age?

YES → Call your doctor or clinic within the next few hours.

NO

Is your child having difficulty breathing which does not go away when her nose is cleared?

YES → Turn to page 16 for discussion of breathing problems. Your child has more than a simple cold.

NO

Use a cool-mist humidifier, or a pan of water on top of a radiator (if you have this type of heating) to ease the congestion during sleep.

Do not give your child an antibiotic. Antibiotics are useless against colds, and they are potentially harmful, especially when a leftover prescription is used.

Do not give your child any home remedies or massive doses of vitamins. (Of course, homemade soups are fine.)

There is no reason why your child cannot go outdoors. This will not make her cold worse.

Is your child congested to the point that it is interfering with her feeding (infants) or sleep?

NO

YES

(continued on next page)

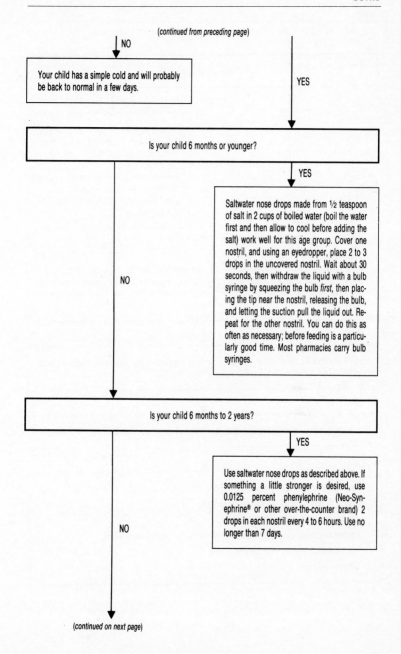

(*continued from preceding page*)

NO

Your child has a simple cold and will probably be back to normal in a few days.

YES

Is your child 6 months or younger?

YES

Saltwater nose drops made from ½ teaspoon of salt in 2 cups of boiled water (boil the water first and then allow to cool before adding the salt) work well for this age group. Cover one nostril, and using an eyedropper, place 2 to 3 drops in the uncovered nostril. Wait about 30 seconds, then withdraw the liquid with a bulb syringe by squeezing the bulb *first*, then placing the tip near the nostril, releasing the bulb, and letting the suction pull the liquid out. Repeat for the other nostril. You can do this as often as necessary; before feeding is a particularly good time. Most pharmacies carry bulb syringes.

NO

Is your child 6 months to 2 years?

YES

Use saltwater nose drops as described above. If something a little stronger is desired, use 0.0125 percent phenylephrine (Neo-Synephrine® or other over-the-counter brand) 2 drops in each nostril every 4 to 6 hours. Use no longer than 7 days.

NO

(*continued on next page*)

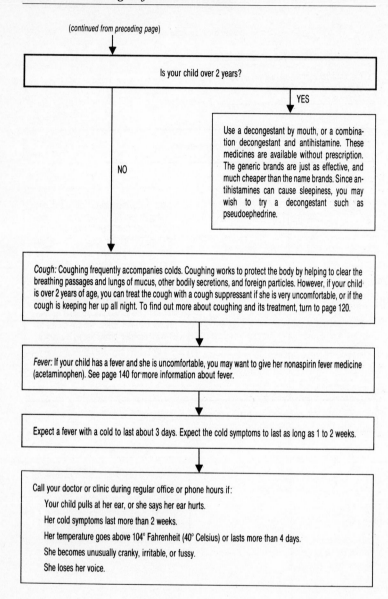

(continued from preceding page)

Is your child over 2 years?

YES

Use a decongestant by mouth, or a combination decongestant and antihistamine. These medicines are available without prescription. The generic brands are just as effective, and much cheaper than the name brands. Since antihistamines can cause sleepiness, you may wish to try a decongestant such as pseudoephedrine.

NO

Cough: Coughing frequently accompanies colds. Coughing works to protect the body by helping to clear the breathing passages and lungs of mucus, other bodily secretions, and foreign particles. However, if your child is over 2 years of age, you can treat the cough with a cough suppressant if she is very uncomfortable, or if the cough is keeping her up all night. To find out more about coughing and its treatment, turn to page 120.

Fever: If your child has a fever and she is uncomfortable, you may want to give her nonaspirin fever medicine (acetaminophen). See page 140 for more information about fever.

Expect a fever with a cold to last about 3 days. Expect the cold symptoms to last as long as 1 to 2 weeks.

Call your doctor or clinic during regular office or phone hours if:

Your child pulls at her ear, or she says her ear hurts.

Her cold symptoms last more than 2 weeks.

Her temperature goes above 104° Fahrenheit (40° Celsius) or lasts more than 4 days.

She becomes unusually cranky, irritable, or fussy.

She loses her voice.

More about Colds

Colds are a very common type of infection which people can get at any age. Infants and children get more colds than adults do because their defenses against infection are not fully developed.

There are over a hundred different types of viruses that can cause colds. Viruses are a type of germ. Common folklore has it that colds are caused by exposure to cold weather. This is not true. Colds are caused by close contact with other people who are carrying one of the cold viruses.

In the early phase of a cold, the discharge from the nose is clear, thin, and runny. After several days, this thickens and causes congestion. Other symptoms include fever, mild sore throat, sneezing, coughing, and headache. Fever with a cold usually lasts less than three days, while the other cold symptoms can last up to two weeks.

There is no cure for the common cold. Vitamin C has no proven effect in reducing either the number or severity of colds. Tonsils and adenoids do not cause colds, and removing them will not change a person's susceptibility to colds. In fact, tonsils and adenoids are part of the body's defenses for fighting off colds and other infections. They may appear large in children not because they are infected but because they grow at a faster rate than the rest of the body until about 13 or 14 years of age. To learn more about tonsillectomies, turn to Chapter 37, "Sore Throats and Tonsillitis."

Too Many Colds

Parents are often concerned because their child seems to have a cold that lasts "all winter." Preschool children average *eight colds a year*. Since each of these colds can last one to two weeks this makes for between *two and four months' worth* of cold symptoms a year! The peak time for colds is September, when children start back to school, share their germs with their new classmates, and bring the germs home. A child who is active and is growing and gaining weight normally does not get too many colds.

Conditions That Seem to Be Colds

There are two conditions that can seem to be colds, but actually are not: hay fever and asthma.

HAY FEVER

One out of every ten people, including children, suffers from hay fever. Hay fever is actually an allergy which causes irritation to the nose and eyes. Unlike a cold, it is not caused by an infection. Symptoms of hay fever include runny and stuffy nose, itchy eyes, tearing, frequent sniffling and rubbing of the nose, and itching of the top of the mouth. Despite its name, there is no fever associated with hay fever.

Hay fever can occur year-round in people who are allergic to such things as house dust and molds. The symptoms usually worsen in the winter, when homes are dustier, especially if forced-air heating is used.

Seasonal hay fever is caused by pollen, which is spread by the wind. Tree pollens are in the air in late winter and early spring. Grass pollens appear in spring and early summer. Weed pollens appear in late summer and early fall.

There are many different ways to treat hay fever. It is best to talk to your doctor or clinic if you suspect your child has hay fever. Sometimes it is necessary to have your child see an allergist and undergo skin tests. The medical term for hay fever is *allergic rhinitis*.

Asthma

Chronic nighttime cough and frequent colds can be the early signs or the only signs of asthma. Snoring and mouth breathing are also often present. Asthma is a problem that affects the breathing passages of the lungs. Turn to Chapter 2, "Breathing Problems," to learn more about asthma.

20. *Constipation*

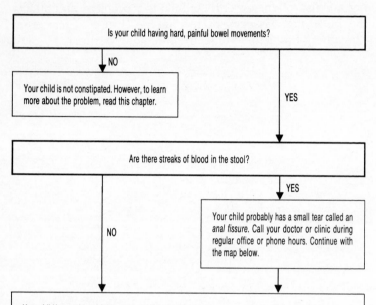

Is your child having hard, painful bowel movements?

NO

Your child is not constipated. However, to learn more about the problem, read this chapter.

YES

Are there streaks of blood in the stool?

YES

Your child probably has a small tear called an *anal fissure*. Call your doctor or clinic during regular office or phone hours. Continue with the map below.

NO

Your child is constipated. It is a problem which should not concern you greatly. It will almost certainly respond to a few simple measures. Try the following for 2 or 3 days:

Younger infants (under 2 months):
Call your doctor or clinic during regular office or phone hours.

Infants (2 months to 1 year):
Add 1 tablespoon of corn syrup to every other 8-ounce bottle of formula. Give one extra feeding of water a day: 2 to 4 ounces for small infants under 6 months, 8 ounces per day for older infants. You can also use gentle rectal stimulation with a rectal thermometer once or twice a day.

Older infants and young toddlers (1 to 2 years):
8 ounces of apple, orange, or prune juice a day, and 8 extra ounces of water a day. Give fruits and vegetables, except bananas. Avoid cheese.

Children over 2 years:
Give fresh fruits and vegetables, except for bananas, twice a day. Give fresh fruit or vegetable juices twice a day. Encourage your child to drink water. Avoid cheese.

(continued on next page)

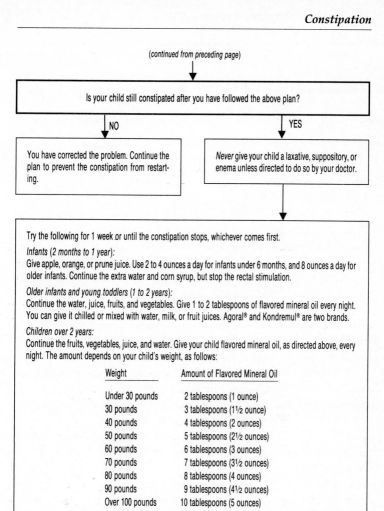

(continued from preceding page)

Is your child still constipated after you have followed the above plan?

NO

You have corrected the problem. Continue the plan to prevent the constipation from restarting.

YES

Never give your child a laxative, suppository, or enema unless directed to do so by your doctor.

Try the following for 1 week or until the constipation stops, whichever comes first.

Infants (2 months to 1 year):
Give apple, orange, or prune juice. Use 2 to 4 ounces a day for infants under 6 months, and 8 ounces a day for older infants. Continue the extra water and corn syrup, but stop the rectal stimulation.

Older infants and young toddlers (1 to 2 years):
Continue the water, juice, fruits, and vegetables. Give 1 to 2 tablespoons of flavored mineral oil every night. You can give it chilled or mixed with water, milk, or fruit juices. Agoral® and Kondremul® are two brands.

Children over 2 years:
Continue the fruits, vegetables, juice, and water. Give your child flavored mineral oil, as directed above, every night. The amount depends on your child's weight, as follows:

Weight	Amount of Flavored Mineral Oil
Under 30 pounds	2 tablespoons (1 ounce)
30 pounds	3 tablespoons (1½ ounce)
40 pounds	4 tablespoons (2 ounces)
50 pounds	5 tablespoons (2½ ounces)
60 pounds	6 tablespoons (3 ounces)
70 pounds	7 tablespoons (3½ ounces)
80 pounds	8 tablespoons (4 ounces)
90 pounds	9 tablespoons (4½ ounces)
Over 100 pounds	10 tablespoons (5 ounces)

Do not worry that these amounts are more than what is suggested on the bottle. Mineral oil is extremely safe and non-habit-forming. It only works well at these dosages.

Is your child still constipated?

NO

YES

(continued on next page)

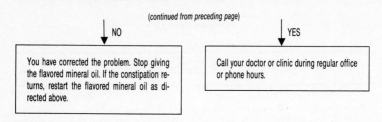

More about Constipation

Constipation is a problem that often worries parents, sometimes needlessly. It is not necessary for your child to have one bowel movement at the same time every day. It is not necessarily healthier to be "regular." As long as your child is having soft or pasty bowel movements at least once every two to four days, he is not constipated.

Some parents are concerned because they think it is dangerous for stool to stay inside their child. Understand that a child cannot be poisoned by his own stool inside his digestive system.

It is best to take a calm and relaxed approach to bowel habits. Too much attention paid to this function can make matters worse. If you put too much pressure on your child to have bowel movements, it becomes a struggle between you and the child. This is a struggle which the child will almost always win, because it is much easier for him to hold back his bowel movements than it is for you to make him have one. The same principles apply to toilet training, which should not start until your child is at least 2 years old—unless he definitely indicates that he is ready.

Hard, painful bowel movements can be a problem, however. A hard movement can tear the anus (the opening through which bowel movements pass). The tears, called *anal fissures,* are small and difficult to see. Suspect them if you see small streaks of blood in the bowel movement. These tears can be quite painful and can make children afraid of having more bowel movements, which only worsens the constipation.

Anal fissures require prompt medical attention, but they are not an emergency. It is a good idea to contact a doctor within a day of discovering blood-streaked stools. The treatment of an anal fissure usually consists of suppositories to loosen stools and frequent warm, soapy baths to soak the tender area.

Infants at times use great effort to produce a bowel movement. They squeeze very hard and turn red in the face. This does not mean they are in pain. Infants have less-developed belly muscles, and it takes extra effort to move their bowels. Do not worry about your infant *unless* the bowel movements are hard, occur less than once every three days, or have streaks of blood in them.

Parents are often very concerned about the different colors of stool, especially in infants. It is normal for stool to change color depending on what is eaten. Newborn infants have dark green, sticky stool. This soon changes to green-yellow, seedy, pasty stool. As children grow, their stool comes to resemble that of adults. A sudden change in the color of feces is almost always caused by ingestion of some different-colored food.

Never give your child a laxative, suppository, or enema unless directed to do so by your doctor. The use of stool-softeners is the best and the safest way to treat constipation. Stool-softeners can be obtained without prescription and are not habit-forming. Mineral oil is the best and safest stool-softener available. It works by coating the stool in a slippery covering. Flavored mineral oil tastes something like a milkshake; most children will drink it without complaining.

21. *Coughing*

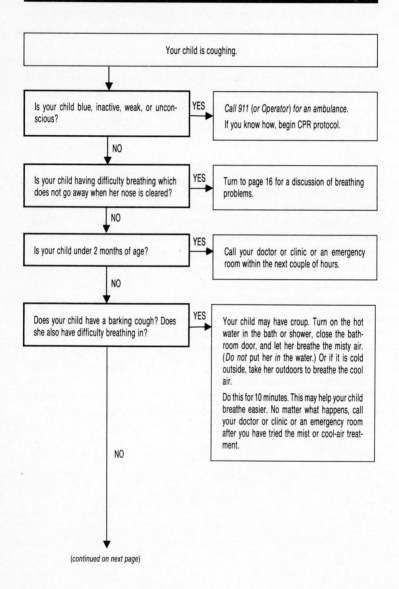

Your child is coughing.

Is your child blue, inactive, weak, or unconscious?

YES → *Call 911 (or Operator) for an ambulance.* If you know how, begin CPR protocol.

NO

Is your child having difficulty breathing which does not go away when her nose is cleared?

YES → Turn to page 16 for a discussion of breathing problems.

NO

Is your child under 2 months of age?

YES → Call your doctor or clinic or an emergency room within the next couple of hours.

NO

Does your child have a barking cough? Does she also have difficulty breathing in?

YES → Your child may have croup. Turn on the hot water in the bath or shower, close the bathroom door, and let her breathe the misty air. (*Do not* put her *in* the water.) Or if it is cold outside, take her outdoors to breathe the cool air.

Do this for 10 minutes. This may help your child breathe easier. No matter what happens, call your doctor or clinic or an emergency room after you have tried the mist or cool-air treatment.

NO

(continued on next page)

(*continued from preceding page*)

If your child is under 2 years of age, she should not be given a cough suppressant, except when a physician so directs. This is because younger children depend more on the protective clearing action of coughing. At this age it is dangerous to block the coughing reflex.

If your child is *over* 2 years of age, you can treat the cough with a cough suppressant if your child is very uncomfortable, or if the cough is keeping her up all night.

You can use any brand of cough medicine as long as it contains dextromethorphan. Most brands will have *DM* in the name of the product to indicate they contain dextromethorphan. The generic brands of cough suppressant are just as effective and are much cheaper than the name brands. You can buy cough suppressants without a prescription.

Check the dosage on the box of the cough medicine. Short-acting cough medicines are given every 4 to 6 hours. Longer-acting preparations are given every 8 to 12 hours.

Do not give your child an antibiotic unless directed to do so by your doctor. Antibiotics are useless against most coughs. They are potentially harmful, particularly when a leftover prescription is used.

Do not give your child any home remedies or massive doses of vitamins. (Of course, homemade soups are fine.)

Does your child also have a cold?

NO

Call your doctor during regular office or phone hours if:

Your child loses her voice.

The cough lasts more than a few days.

You have any questions or concerns.

YES

Do not be concerned if the cough stays with the cold for 1 to 2 weeks.

Turn to page 110 to learn more about colds.

Call your doctor or clinic during regular office or phone hours if:

The coughing lasts more than two weeks.

Your child has multiple episodes of night-time coughing.

Your child loses her voice.

You have any questions or concerns.

More about Coughing

Coughing commonly affects both children and adults. It is caused by anything that irritates the respiratory passages enough to trigger the cough reflex. This is a protective reflex that helps to clear out substances that can harm the lungs.

The usual cause of a cough is the common cold, in which there is excessive mucus production. The mucus triggers the cough reflex. Other common causes of coughing include foreign objects, such as food that goes down the "wrong pipe"; noxious fumes such as cigarette smoke; and asthma. The only symptom of asthma may be frequent bouts of nighttime coughing (discussed in Chapter 2, "Breathing Problems").

Croup (rhymes with *soup*) is an illness of young children which produces a characteristic barking cough. It responds particularly well to very humid or cold air. Croup also is discussed in detail in Chapter 2.

A child can be made very uncomfortable by coughing, especially if it keeps her awake at night. The coughing is often quite worrisome to parents. It is reasonable to want to try and stop the coughing and relieve your child's suffering. It should be kept in mind, however, that coughing by itself is not dangerous. It is a symptom of a problem.

As described above, coughing is a protective response by the body. Suppressing a cough with cough medicine not only reduces this protective clearing action but also may mask a more serious underlying problem. It is particularly important that young children under the age of 2 years *not be given* cough medicines unless a physician so directs. Young children's lungs are more sensitive, and are thus more dependent on the protection coughing provides.

For these reasons cough medicines must be used with care. It is fine to use a cough-suppressing medicine for a brief time, as directed on the map, with an older child who has a cold. Any other use should first be cleared with your doctor. Keep in mind that cough medicines do not always work well. This can be annoying, but it should not worry you. Also, the cough suppressant at best will reduce the intensity and frequency of the cough; it will not speed recovery.

22. *Diaper Rash*

Your infant has diaper rash.

Don't feel guilty; *all* babies get diaper rash at one time or another.

Don't frustrate yourself trying to get rid of all patches of diaper rash.

Diaper rash is not a dangerous condition.

Try the measures listed below.

Keep your infant clean and dry with frequent diaper changes.

Avoid rubber pants when possible.

Keep the diapers off as much as possible.

Do not use petroleum jelly. This only keeps the baby's skin wet and moist—conditions which promote diaper rash.

Use some type of baby powder to keep the skin dry.

Apply an ointment containing vitamins A and D to the rash 3 to 4 times a day. Continue its use on the baby's bottom even after the rash clears up.

Call your doctor or clinic during regular office or phone hours if:

The rash gets beefy-red.

You have any questions or concerns.

More about Diaper Rash

Diaper rash is the most common rash of infancy. Almost all infants will get diaper rash at one time or another. It is caused by several factors. To begin with, infants have delicate skin. Contact with urine and feces, which contain skin-irritating chemicals, can cause a rash, especially after prolonged contact. Diarrhea can trigger an outbreak of diaper rash or worsen a preexisting rash. Diaper rash is generally worse in the winter, when diapers have to stay on longer and diarrhea is more common.

The measures mentioned on the map will help you control your baby's diaper rash. The goal should be to keep the rash at a minimum, since total elimination is often not possible. Most infants will have a small patch of rash in the genital region that comes and goes.

Certain recent studies suggest that paper diapers containing absorbent chemicals may be superior to standard paper or cloth diapers in preventing diaper rash. However, the most important measure continues to be keeping your infant clean and dry with frequent diaper changes.

Sometimes a diaper rash will become covered with a yeast infection which gives the rash a raw, beefy-red appearance. This is best treated by a prescription antifungal cream. The cream is applied three to four times a day for 10 to 14 days. *Thrush,* which is a yeast infection of the mouth (see Chapter 31, "Newborn Babies"), can at times trigger a yeast infection of the diapered area. Treatment requires both a cream to the diapered area and liquid in the mouth.

23. *Diarrhea*

Diarrhea usually starts suddenly. Your child will have loose, watery stools. He may be irritable, have a fever, and begin vomiting.

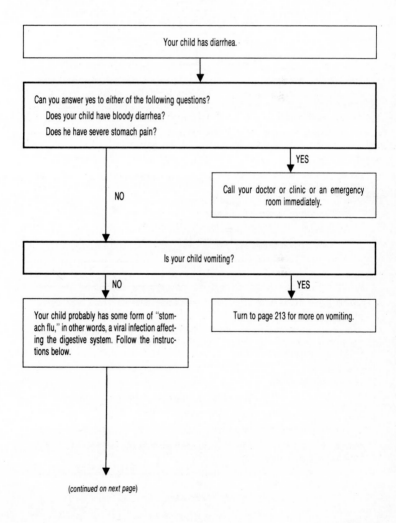

Your child has diarrhea.

Can you answer yes to *either* of the following questions?
Does your child have bloody diarrhea?
Does he have severe stomach pain?

YES

NO

Call your doctor or clinic or an emergency room immediately.

Is your child vomiting?

NO

YES

Your child probably has some form of "stomach flu," in other words, a viral infection affecting the digestive system. Follow the instructions below.

Turn to page 213 for more on vomiting.

(continued on next page)

(continued from preceding page)

Give your child clear liquids which are *not* dietetic or sugar-free. *Do not* give milk or orange juice, as these tend to upset the stomach. *Do not* give solid foods.

Under 1 year of age:
Use commercially prepared clear fluids such as Lytren® or Pedialyte® for infants. Feed your infant every 2 to 3 hours. Offer him as much as he takes in a regular feeding. It is fine to give several extra feedings per day.

Over 1 year of age:
Use water, flat ginger ale, apple juice (half-strength for younger children), and other clear fruit juices and fruit drinks, Gatorade®, Jell-o®, clear soup broth, and ice desserts. Make sure your child drinks every 1 to 2 hours.

You may give your child nonaspirin fever medicine (acetaminophen) if he has a fever and seems uncomfortable (see page 143 for the proper dose). You may give antidiarrhea medicine, such as Kaopectate® or similar brand to children over 10 years of age. Check the bottle for proper dose. Otherwise, *do not give your child any medicines,* including aspirin, unless directed to do so by your doctor.

It is very important that you keep giving your child plenty of clear fluids, particularly if he has a fever. Dehydration will result if fluid losses are too great. The warning signs of dehydration in infants and children are:

No urination for 8 to 10 hours   Sunken eyes

Very dry mouth   Extreme sleepiness and difficulty waking up

Call your doctor or clinic or an emergency room immediately if you think your child is becoming dehydrated.

Count the number of stools your child has in a day. If he starts getting better after 24 hours, do the following:

Under 1 year of age:
Start with either half-strength soy-based formula (Prosobee® or Isomil®) or quarter-strength regular formula. Slowly increase the strength of the formula over the next 2 to 3 days. You should not have to continue the soy-based formula for more than 5 to 7 days.

Over 1 year of age:
Begin with the following foods:

Bananas	Bland crackers such as Saltines®	Dry toast
Rice	Carrots (raw or cooked)	
Rice cereal without milk	Peeled apples or applesauce	

Keep giving the clear fluids, but taper the amount as the child gets better. Keep him off milk for 5 to 7 days. Slowly bring him back to a regular diet.

(continued on next page)

(continued from preceding page)

Call your doctor or clinic during regular office or phone hours if:

The number of stools in a day does not decrease after you have given your child clear liquids for 24 to 36 hours.

You have any questions or concerns.

More about Diarrhea

Diarrhea is a very common problem, usually caused by germs called *viruses*. Virally caused diarrhea is usually accompanied by vomiting, mild fever, and other symptoms such as muscle aches and a general run-down feeling. This type of diarrhea is sometimes referred to as a *stomach bug* or *stomach flu*.

The most important thing to keep in mind when your child develops diarrhea is to make sure he does not become dehydrated. This is particularly important in infants. Dehydration follows when the body loses too much fluid. Don't worry if your child goes several days without solid food; this will not harm him. The preceding map instructs you in how to treat diarrhea and how to spot the early signs of dehydration.

Dehydration is easily avoided by giving the child plenty of fluids. Full recovery from diarrhea usually takes at least four to seven days.

After an illness with diarrhea, the digestive system is sensitive to milk and milk-based formulas. For this reason, milk-based formulas have to be thinned for infants; older children should avoid milk products for several days after a diarrhea episode. A soy-based formula can also be used for an infant who has an episode of diarrhea.

It is unusual for diarrhea to last for more than a week or two. If your child develops persistent diarrhea, he needs the doctor's attention. Chronic diarrhea may require certain medicines or special diets.

24. *Earaches*

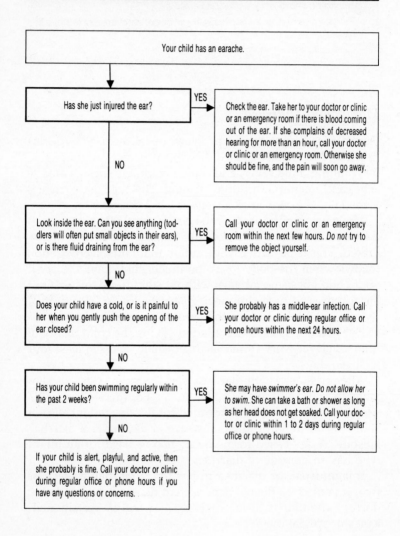

Your child has an earache.

Has she just injured the ear?

YES → Check the ear. Take her to your doctor or clinic or an emergency room if there is blood coming out of the ear. If she complains of decreased hearing for more than an hour, call your doctor or clinic or an emergency room. Otherwise she should be fine, and the pain will soon go away.

NO

Look inside the ear. Can you see anything (toddlers will often put small objects in their ears), or is there fluid draining from the ear?

YES → Call your doctor or clinic or an emergency room within the next few hours. *Do not* try to remove the object yourself.

NO

Does your child have a cold, or is it painful to her when you gently push the opening of the ear closed?

YES → She probably has a middle-ear infection. Call your doctor or clinic during regular office or phone hours within the next 24 hours.

NO

Has your child been swimming regularly within the past 2 weeks?

YES → She may have *swimmer's ear. Do not allow her to swim.* She can take a bath or shower as long as her head does not get soaked. Call your doctor or clinic within 1 to 2 days during regular office or phone hours.

NO

If your child is alert, playful, and active, then she probably is fine. Call your doctor or clinic during regular office or phone hours if you have any questions or concerns.

More about Earaches

Earaches can be caused by several different conditions. The most common cause of earache is infection of either the ear canal or the middle ear. Other causes are ear injuries and small objects trapped inside the ear canal.

An illustration of the ear in cross section is provided below. The *outer ear* is the part of the ear you can hold with your hand. The *ear canal* is the tubular passage between the outer ear and the *eardrum*. The *middle ear* is on the other side of the eardrum. *Eustachian* (pronounced: you *sta*tion) *tubes* act as pressure valves to protect the eardrum. They cause the "pop" when you yawn during a plane landing or long elevator descent. The *inner ear* is the innermost part of the ear, which contains the sensors of sound and balance.

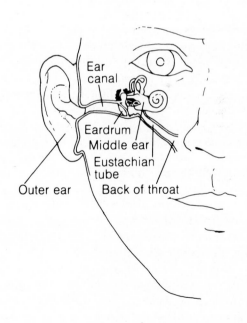

MIDDLE-EAR INFECTIONS

Middle-ear infections are very common among children. They almost always occur with colds. It is easy to tell if an older child has an earache. It is not so easy, however, with babies and toddlers, because they cannot tell you where they hurt. Sometimes an infant will pull or rub on the painful ear or on both ears. More likely than not, however, the only sign of ear problems in infants will be fever and irritability. The medical term for a middle-ear infection is *otitis media* (pronounced: oh *tight* us *meed* ee uh).

Otitis media is diagnosed by the appearance of the eardrum. Your doctor will look into your child's ear canal and visualize the eardrum with a special hand-held light. An infected middle ear will cause the eardrum to look red and bulging. The eardrum normally moves easily. If there is increased fluid in the ear because of an infection, or a resolving infection, the drum will be less mobile.

Movement of the eardrum can be checked by an attachment on the hand-held light which changes the air pressure in the ear canal while the doctor checks the drum for movement. A machine called a *tympanometer* (pronounced: tim-*pan*-ah-mēt-ur) can also check for fluid by measuring pressure changes in the ear canal. An earmuff-appearing device is placed over your child's ear. This is a safe and painless test.

The exact cause of middle-ear infections in children is not known. Research shows they may develop because the eustachian tubes of infants and children close easily. When a tube is closed off during a cold, the situation is ripe for a middle-ear infection. Adults, whose eustachian tubes are more rigid, rarely get middle-ear infections.

Middle-ear infections are caused by bacteria; thus, we can treat them with antibiotics. An antibiotic is given by mouth for a week to 10 days. Eardrops with a mild painkiller will often make a very painful ear feel better. Aspirin or nonaspirin pain and fever medicine (acetaminophen) by mouth also work well. It is sometimes necessary to switch to a second or even a third antibiotic if the infection does not clear up.

A middle-ear infection that occurs quickly or goes untreated sometimes causes the eardrum to perforate; the mucus and pus produced during the infection cause enough pressure to tear the eardrum.

Repeated ear infections are a relatively common problem for young children. One method of treatment is to place small plastic tubes in the child's ear. The technical name for this procedure is tympanostomy (pronounced: tim pan *oss* toe me). It is performed by an ENT (ear, nose, and throat) surgeon in an operating room under general anesthesia. Tympanostomy tubes supposedly work by letting air into the middle ear.

Tympanostomy is very popular, but its value is unproven. Although research is being done constantly, no study has shown that the tubes work better than antibiotics. I feel that in many situations tubes are unnecessary. The operation carries the risks associated with general anesthesia, and the tubes sometimes scar the eardrum. There are certain children who *will* benefit from tubes, however. Since this is a very controversial subject, it is best to discuss it with your pediatrician or family doctor.

SWIMMER'S EAR

Swimmer's ear is an infection of the skin that lines the ear canal. It is caused by a type of bacteria that lives in water and is commonly found in pools and lakes. Swimmer's ear is treated by eardrops for one to two weeks. Swimming should be discontinued for at least one week, longer if symptoms persist. It is OK to bathe or shower your child as long as her head does not get soaked.

Infection of the ear canal can happen also when a scratch or scab inside the ear canal becomes infected. The infection has the same symptoms as swimmer's ear, and is treated in the same way.

The medical term for an infected ear canal or swimmer's ear is *otitis externa* (pronounced: oh *tight* us ex *turn* ah).

FOREIGN OBJECTS IN THE EAR

Infants and toddlers are well known for putting small objects in their ears. Unless the object is sticking out and is easily removed, *do not* try to remove it yourself. The ear canal bleeds easily, so care must be taken. A doctor or other medical professional will usually be able to remove the object either by injecting water into the ear or by using forceps. In rare cases, surgery may be necessary.

Routine Ear Cleaning

Ears, like modern ovens, are self-cleaning. It is not necessary and is potentially dangerous to use cotton-tipped ear-cleaning devices. If you feel you must clean your child's ears, let warm water run gently into them during a bath or shower. In rare instances, a wax plug may build up to the point of being painful. This condition is best treated by having your doctor irrigate the ear with warm water from a syringe, or you may be able to treat it at home by using special drops which gradually dissolve the wax.

25. *Feeding Babies and Young Children*

Nothing can be more intimidating than your first attempts at feeding a young baby. Questions such as the following invariably arise: Is he eating enough? Is he eating too much? Is he burping enough? Is he eating too soon? Is he going too long between feedings? As you get to know your baby and his eating style, you will be able to tell most of the time what he wants. Trust your judgment, and give yourself credit. Don't be afraid to follow your intuition and assessment of your baby's needs.

Do not try to force a rigid feeding schedule on your baby. Don't worry if he doesn't finish the entire bottle. A baby lets you know when he is finished eating because he loses interest in the breast or bottle. He keeps turning away from the breast or nipple when it is placed in his mouth, or he simply falls asleep.

The general guidelines for feeding babies and young children are given below. Since every baby is a little different, don't be surprised if your feeding schedule and approach varies somewhat from these guidelines. If at any point you have questions and concerns about feeding your baby, consult your doctor or clinic. A baby who gains weight properly is being fed properly.

Feeding Babies under 1 Year of Age

From birth to 6 months of age, babies should either be breast-fed or be fed commercial formula. Breast-fed babies should receive a supplement containing fluoride and vitamins A, D, and C. A prescription is required for vitamin and mineral supplements containing fluoride. Babies fed commercial formula do not require a vitamin or mineral supplement. However, fluoride supplementation is necessary for bottle-fed babies if your water supply is not fluoridated. For formula-fed babies most pediatricians recommend that commercial formula without extra iron be used for the first 2 months of life, thereafter commercial formula fortified with iron is recommended. Iron supplementation is necessary for infants over 6 months of age who are exclusively breast-fed and are not receiving iron from other sources, such as cereal.

Babies do not require solid foods before 4 to 6 months of age. In fact, babies under 4 to 6 months cannot safely swallow solid food; they may choke on it, causing serious lung and breathing problems.

Infants under 3 months of age eat every 2½ to 4 hours, with even longer stretches between feedings at night. They generally take 2 to 4 ounces per feeding by 2 weeks of age. This increases to 5 to 6 ounces per feeding by 3 months of age. By 6 months babies will be taking 7 to 8 ounces per feeding, and will be eating four times a day. Breast-fed babies generally eat the same number of times a day as bottle-fed babies, and will spend from 5 to 15 minutes on each breast.

It is advisable to give supplemental water or half-strength apple juice during hot summer weather. Babies with diarrhea will have to be fed differently for a short period of time; see Chapter 23, "Diarrhea," for more details.

BREAST OR BOTTLE FEEDING?

I feel that it is all right to use either of these two methods. Both allow for healthy growth. Families must choose the method that works best for them. With breast feeding a bottle of formula can be given from time to time as a supplement. And, in fact, giving a supplementary bottle makes weaning easier, and it allows fathers to become intimately involved in the feeding process.

The most important aspect of feeding babies is to make the

experience intimate, pleasant, and enjoyable for everyone involved. This fosters an emotionally nourishing bond between you and your baby, and it can be accomplished with either bottle or breast feeding. If you have the option, breast milk, with its special properties is probably the better choice, but formula is a perfectly acceptable alternative.

TYPES OF COMMERCIAL FORMULA

There are two basic types of formula: milk-sugar-based formula, and soy-based formula. *Lactose* is the scientific name for milk sugar. Unless directed by your doctor to do otherwise, you should start your baby with a commercial lactose-based formula containing iron. Premature babies may require special formula. Doctors often recommend switching to a soy-based formula if feeding difficulties develop or for a short period after a bout of diarrhea.

BURPING

A breast-fed baby should be burped when he is changed from one breast to the other and at the end of the feeding. With some infants burping has to be more frequent. Small formula-fed babies should be burped after every 1 to 2 ounces, older babies after every 4 to 8 ounces. At least one and usually two burps should be produced. Your baby may not always burp; this is fine if he is comfortable. Use your hand to give rapid, gentle pats on your baby's back. Your baby can be held in three different positions to be burped:

1. Lying against your shoulder
2. Lying on your lap, face down, with your hand under his belly
3. Sitting on your lap with your hand against his belly

Walking with your baby lying against your shoulder as you burp him is often very effective. It sometimes takes 5 to 10 minutes to get a burp, so be patient.

135

Positions for Burping a Baby

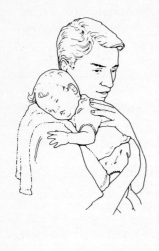

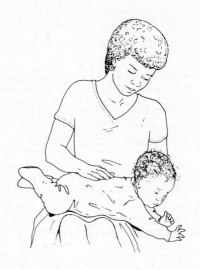

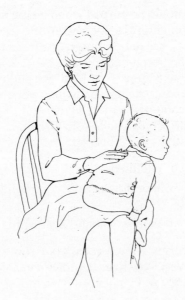

Adding Solid Food

Four to six months of age is the time to start feeding your baby solid food. Start with single-grain infant cereals such as rice, barley, or oats. Introduce one kind of cereal at a time. Begin with 1 or 2 tablespoons of cereal mixed with enough formula or 2 percent milk to make the cereal thin and runny. Start with one feeding a day and increase to two feedings a day, giving 3 to 4 tablespoons maximum per feeding. Feed your baby with a baby spoon. *Do not* add cereal to your baby's formula; this may cause him to choke. *Do not* add salt, sugar, or honey to the cereal.

Over time you may add strained vegetables and then fruits to your baby's diet. Begin with carrots, squash, green beans, or peas. Introduce one vegetable at a time. Start with 2 or 3 tablespoons, and gradually increase to ¼ to ½ cup a day. After your baby has gotten used to vegetables, you may add strained fruits such as bananas, peaches, applesauce, plumbs, pears, or apricots. As with vegetables, begin with 2 or 3 tablespoons and gradually increase to ¼ to ½ cup per day. Use commercially prepared vegetables and fruits, or pre-pare your own. When preparing your own, make sure to peel and pit the fruit or vegetable, then blend or puree it.

A baby between 10 to 12 months of age should be eating three or four meals a day. Encourage your baby to eat finely chopped, soft table foods. Feed him slowly. There is really no need to buy "junior foods," but you may find them more convenient. It is most economical to give the toddler what you eat for dinner as long as the food is soft and finely chopped. At 10 to 12 months you may also add eggs to your child's diet.

Weaning from the Breast

When to start weaning is a very individual decision. About half the time infants start weaning themselves around 5 to 9 months of age as they take more solids. This is fine. Most women will choose to wean their infants from 3 to 12 months of age. It is generally not advisable to breast-feed an infant beyond the age of 1 year since babies become too emotionally dependent on their mothers, and babies' many teeth at this age could make it too painful for their mothers.

Weaning from the breast should be done gradually. Start by eliminating one breast feeding, either the late morning or early afternoon feeding, and substitute a bottle or cup of 2 percent milk (or formula for babies under 9 months). After a few days, substitute a bottle or cup for another feeding. If you run into difficulty, hold off on any further weaning for several days and then resume the weaning process. Gradual weaning should allow the breasts to become adjusted painlessly to lower milk demands.

Weaning is often more easily accomplished by having the baby's father, or anyone else except the mother, give the bottle. This is because the mother's breasts provide strong emotional, physical, and nutritive stimulation to the baby, who at this point is perfectly content with the arrangement. Having the mother's breasts "out of sight and out of mind" can be very helpful. Offer the bottle a half hour before the usual nursing time so your baby does not feel additionally stressed at a time when he is most hungry.

WHEN TO STOP COMMERCIAL FORMULA

Babies should be switched from formula to 2 percent milk at between 6 to 12 months of age. Most pediatricians recommend switching at about 9 months. Usually the switch can be made suddenly with little problem.

Be sure to give your baby 2 percent milk, not skim or whole milk. Skim milk does not contain enough fat. Whole cow's milk should probably never be given to anyone, except baby cattle. This may be surprising, but it is true. And although it will be disputed by the dairy industry, the medical evidence is not on their side. Individuals who drink whole milk on a regular basis risk hardening of the arteries, because whole milk contains large quantities of saturated fats.

Feeding Children Over 1 Year of Age

By 1 year of age your infant should be eating three or four meals a day. He should be drinking no more than 32 ounces a day of 2 percent milk. Water and juice can be given freely.

It is not necessary to give vitamin or mineral supplements to children over 1 year of age, except for fluoride if your water supply is not fluoridated. A well-balanced diet should provide all the necessary nutrients. Do not worry if your toddler has erratic eating patterns. This is very normal at this age. Toddlers will often pick at their food for several meals, then consume an almost adult-sized meal.

Foods that Can Cause Choking

Certain foods should be avoided in younger children. Under 6 or 7 years of age children have not yet developed fully coordinated swallowing and chewing abilities, and they can choke easily on these foods. The foods to avoid include:

Hard and large pieces of food: especially hard candy and large pieces of meat.

Peanuts, chunky peanut butter, bacon, and popcorn: Peanuts are very slippery and can pass easily into a child's windpipe. Bacon breaks into small slivers which can travel easily into the lungs. Popcorn is very light; it, too, can be sucked easily into a child's lungs.

Gum: If swallowed, can cause choking in young children.

26. *Fever*

You cannot tell if your child has a fever merely by checking to see if she feels hot to the touch. You must take her temperature. (See the instructions for use of thermometers, page 73.) A fever is present when there is a temperature by mouth or rectum of 101° Fahrenheit (38.3° Celsius) or greater. *F* and *C* are the abbreviations for Fahrenheit and Celsius.

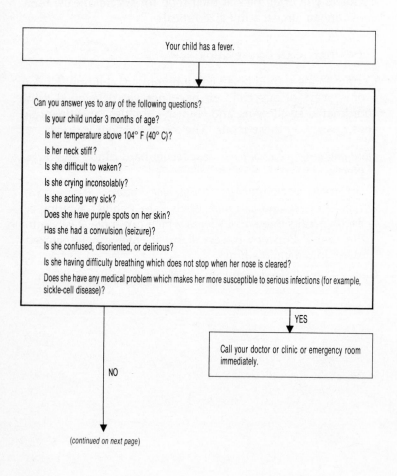

Your child has a fever.

Can you answer yes to *any* of the following questions?

Is your child under 3 months of age?

Is her temperature above 104° F (40° C)?

Is her neck stiff?

Is she difficult to waken?

Is she crying inconsolably?

Is she acting very sick?

Does she have purple spots on her skin?

Has she had a convulsion (seizure)?

Is she confused, disoriented, or delirious?

Is she having difficulty breathing which does not stop when her nose is cleared?

Does she have any medical problem which makes her more susceptible to serious infections (for example, sickle-cell disease)?

YES

Call your doctor or clinic or emergency room immediately.

NO

(continued on next page)

(continued from preceding page)

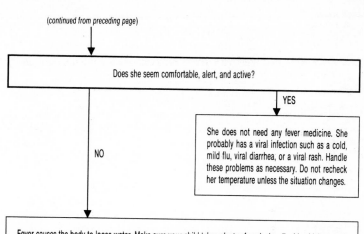

Does she seem comfortable, alert, and active?

YES

She does not need any fever medicine. She probably has a viral infection such as a cold, mild flu, viral diarrhea, or a viral rash. Handle these problems as necessary. Do not recheck her temperature unless the situation changes.

NO

Fever causes the body to loose water. Make sure your child takes *plenty of cool, clear liquids* which are not dietetic or sugar-free. *Do not* give orange juice or milk, as they tend to upset the stomach. *Do not* give solid foods.

Under 1 year of age:
Use commercially prepared clear fluids such as Lytren® and Pedialyte® for infants. Feed your infant every 2 to 3 hours. Offer her as much as she takes in a regular feeding. It is fine to give several extra feedings per day.

Over 1 year of age:
Use water, flat ginger ale, apple juice (half-strength for younger children), and other clear fruit juices and fruit drinks, Gatorade®, Jell-o®, clear soup broth, and ice desserts. Make sure your child drinks every 1 to 2 hours. Do not worry if she does not take any solid foods for a few days, but liquids *must* be taken to avoid dehydration.

Dehydration occurs when the body loses too much water. The warning signs of dehydration in infants and children are:

No urination for 8 to 10 hours   Sunken eyes

Very dry mouth   Extreme sleepiness and difficulty waking up

Call your doctor or clinic or an emergency room immediately if you think your child is becoming dehydrated.

Aspirin should *not* be given to a child with fever, because of the risk of Reye's syndrome (see page 191).

You may give your child nonaspirin fever medicine (acetaminophen).

The dosages for acetaminophen are given following this map.

(continued on next page)

(continued from preceding page)

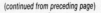

Check your child's temperature every 4 to 6 hours. You may give nonaspirin fever medicine (acetaminophen) for a temperature of 101° F (38.3° C) or greater.

Keep your child *lightly clothed at all times*. Overbundling keeps in body heat and can be dangerous. Your child needs only an undershirt and diapers or underpants.

Keep your child's room cool and well ventilated. The room should be no warmer than 70° F. Keep the window open a crack.

You can give sponge baths but use only lukewarm water. *Do not* use rubbing alcohol.

Call your doctor or clinic during regular office or phone hours if:

Burning or pain occurs with urination.

The fever lasts for more than 24 hours without an obvious cause.

The fever goes away for more than 24 hours and then returns.

The fever lasts for more than 3 days.

You have any questions or concerns.

More about Fever

Fever in a child is a cause of great concern to parents. It is important to remember that fever is not a disease but is most often the sign of an infection.

Fever most often is caused by germs called *viruses,* the type of germs that cause colds and the flu, for example. When fever results from more serious infections, like those caused by bacteria, then it can be a helpful warning signal.

Fever is caused by the body reacting to chemicals produced by germs. It is the germs causing the fever, not the fever itself, that can be dangerous. In fact, research shows that in certain ways fever may help the body fight infection. For example, white blood cells attack germs more efficiently at higher temperatures.

It is important to know when your child's fever is a danger signal. The map for this chapter tells when the fever is a signal to seek medical attention for your child.

Fever causes the body to loose more water than usual, especially in infants and young children. That is why it is so important to make sure a feverish child drinks plenty of fluids. If your child's appetite is poor, it is not a cause for alarm as long as she is taking enough fluids.

Fever can cause discomfort, headache, muscle aches, and irritability. You treat a fever primarily to make your child more comfortable, but you should not overtreat a fever. Nonaspirin fever medicine (acetaminophen) is safe when used properly, but like any medicine it is not entirely free of risk.

A Word about Aspirin and Fever

Research has linked Reye's syndrome (see Chapter 36) with aspirin given to children who have the flu or chicken pox. The cause of this relationship is not presently known. Reye's syndrome is not caused by the aspirin itself. It is completely safe to give aspirin, in the proper dosage, to children who do not have influenza or chicken pox. And once a child has completely recovered from these diseases, it is safe to give her aspirin when called for.

Many childhood illnesses resemble the flu. For example, it is practically impossible to distinguish a bad cold from a mild case of the flu. For this reason *it is not advisable to treat fever with aspirin in any child under the age of 16.*

Nonaspirin Fever Medicine (Acetaminophen)

The generic term for nonaspirin fever medicine is *acetaminophen* (pronounced: uh set uh *min* uh fin). Tylenol® is one brand, but there are many others. Acetaminophen comes in two liquid strengths: drops and elixir. There are also two tablet strengths: children's chewable tablets and adult tablets. The drops are used only for infants. Ask the druggist to show you the generic acetaminophen; it is no different from the name brands but it can be purchased for a fraction of their cost.

The dosages for nonaspirin fever medicine (acetaminophen) are as follows:

Age	Drops (80 mg per dropper)	Elixir (160 mg per teaspoon)	Tablets (Children's chewable, 80 mg per tablet; adult, 325 mg per tablet)
Under 3 months	*	*	*
3 to 5 months	½ dropper	¼ teaspoon	*
6 to 11 months	1 dropper	½ teaspoon	*
1 to 2 years	1½ droppers	¾ teaspoon	*
2 to 3 years	2 droppers	1 teaspoon	2 chewable
4 to 5 years		1½ teaspoons	3 chewable
6 to 8 years		2 teaspoons	4 chewable or 1 adult
9 to 10 years		2½ teaspoons	5 chewable or 1½ adult
Over 10 years		3 teaspoons	2 adult

* Ask your doctor or clinic.

27. *Fussy Babies*

Your baby is very fussy. He may cry continuously for several hours no matter what you do to comfort him. He may seem hungry even though he has just been fed. He clenches his fists and brings his knees up to his stomach or arches his back. He often quiets down after passing gas. He may be fussiest late in the day. You are probably going crazy and feeling angry, guilty, and frustrated all at the same time.

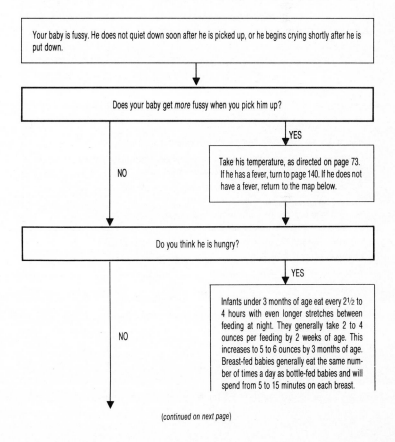

Your baby is fussy. He does not quiet down soon after he is picked up, or he begins crying shortly after he is put down.

Does your baby get *more* fussy when you pick him up?

YES

Take his temperature, as directed on page 73. If he has a fever, turn to page 140. If he does not have a fever, return to the map below.

NO

Do you think he is hungry?

YES

Infants under 3 months of age eat every 2½ to 4 hours with even longer stretches between feeding at night. They generally take 2 to 4 ounces per feeding by 2 weeks of age. This increases to 5 to 6 ounces by 3 months of age. Breast-fed babies generally eat the same number of times a day as bottle-fed babies and will spend from 5 to 15 minutes on each breast.

NO

(continued on next page)

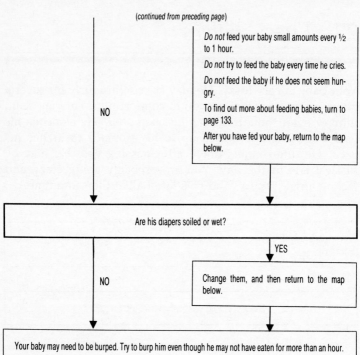

(continued from preceding page)

Do not feed your baby small amounts every ½ to 1 hour.

Do not try to feed the baby every time he cries.

Do not feed the baby if he does not seem hungry.

To find out more about feeding babies, turn to page 133.

After you have fed your baby, return to the map below.

NO

Are his diapers soiled or wet?

YES

NO

Change them, and then return to the map below.

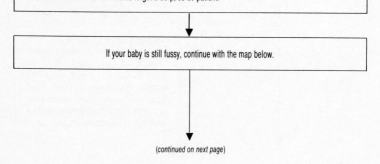

Your baby may need to be burped. Try to burp him even though he may not have eaten for more than an hour.

Small babies should be burped after every 1 to 2 ounces. At least one and usually two burps should be produced. Use your hand to give rapid gentle pats on your baby's back.

Your baby can be held in three different positions to be burped (these positions are illustrated on page 136):

1. Lying against your shoulder
2. Lying on your lap, face down, with your hand under his belly
3. Sitting on your lap with your hand against his belly

Walking with your baby lying against your shoulder as you burp him is often effective.

It sometimes takes 5 to 10 minutes to get a burp, so be patient.

If your baby is still fussy, continue with the map below.

(continued on next page)

146

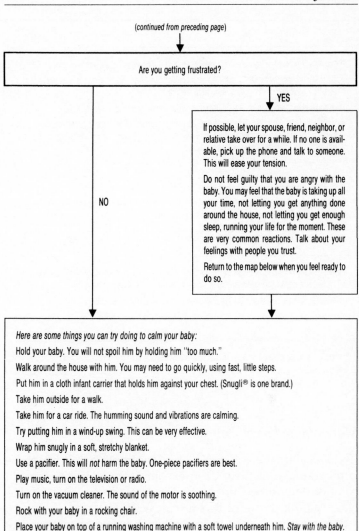

(continued from preceding page)

Are you getting frustrated?

YES

If possible, let your spouse, friend, neighbor, or relative take over for a while. If no one is available, pick up the phone and talk to someone. This will ease your tension.

Do not feel guilty that you are angry with the baby. You may feel that the baby is taking up all your time, not letting you get anything done around the house, not letting you get enough sleep, running your life for the moment. These are very common reactions. Talk about your feelings with people you trust.

Return to the map below when you feel ready to do so.

NO

Here are some things you can try doing to calm your baby:

Hold your baby. You will not spoil him by holding him "too much."

Walk around the house with him. You may need to go quickly, using fast, little steps.

Put him in a cloth infant carrier that holds him against your chest. (Snugli® is one brand.)

Take him outside for a walk.

Take him for a car ride. The humming sound and vibrations are calming.

Try putting him in a wind-up swing. This can be very effective.

Wrap him snugly in a soft, stretchy blanket.

Use a pacifier. This will *not* harm the baby. One-piece pacifiers are best.

Play music, turn on the television or radio.

Turn on the vacuum cleaner. The sound of the motor is soothing.

Rock with your baby in a rocking chair.

Place your baby on top of a running washing machine with a soft towel underneath him. *Stay with the baby.* The motion of the machine quiets some babies.

(continued on next page)

(continued from preceding page)

If your baby is quiet while being held and cries when he is put down, you might try the following:

Wait 5 to 10 minutes after he has fallen asleep before putting him down. This will allow him to get into a deeper sleep before he is disturbed by being moved into the crib.

Have music playing in the room. A wind-up music box or a mobile with music can work well.

As you put the baby down, place one hand flat on the mattress and let his cheek rest on your palm. Gently rock him back and forth with the other hand for 5 to 10 minutes. Slowly withdraw your hand. Stop rocking after 1 or 2 minutes. Leave the room. Keep the music playing.

Leave your baby with your spouse, friend, or relative so you can get out of the house and away from the baby at least 1 hour a day. This is *very important* for your peace of mind.

If at any time you are feeling *overwhelmed* by the situation and are afraid that you are going to hit or otherwise injure the baby, find someone *immediately* to care for the baby for a while.

If no one is available, *call 911 (or Operator)* and tell them you need *Crisis Services.*

If nothing has worked after 1 or 2 weeks, call your doctor or clinic during regular office or phone hours.

More about Fussy Babies

Certain babies are very fussy; this is a simple fact. While there is no shortage of theories to explain it, medical science still has not determined the cause for excessive fussiness in babies. Another term for this fussiness is *colic.*

It is most important to remember that *good parents can have fussy or colicky babies.*

Colic is not more common in breast-fed babies. It is not more common in bottle-fed babies. It is not more common in male babies or in female babies. It is not more common in babies delivered by caesarean section. It is not more common in babies delivered vaginally. Fussy or colicky babies grow as well as noncolicky babies. There is no long-term bad effect of any kind on colicky babies. Nothing you did or didn't do caused the problem.

Probably the worst part of having a fussy baby is your guilt about the negative feelings you're having toward the baby. Here you are, working hard to provide the best for your infant, and he does not seem to care. You have *no time* to get anything done. You are exhausted, frustrated, angry. The baby whom you so anxiously and joyously awaited is now ruining your life—or at least is making it very difficult.

These are all natural feelings. Don't feel guilty. Millions of parents feel the same way. Ventilate. Talk to others about your situation.

Often the thing that makes a baby colicky has nothing to do with the baby himself. Here's an example: a second baby is born into a family with a toddler. The second baby is no more fussy than the first, but now there is less time to quiet the baby because the toddler requires so much attention. Here's another example: a young family lives in an apartment or condo with extremely thin walls, next to an extremely short-tempered widow who has an extremely loud voice and who runs the vacuum cleaner on the wall at 3 in the morning if she thinks the family has made too much noise earlier that day. In these circumstances, even a "perfect angel" may seem colicky.

Colicky babies seem to be more sensitive to certain types of stimulation. The map on the previous pages contains many helpful, specific suggestions. You will notice that *rocking* and *moving* seem to help more than anything else.

Do not worry about letting your baby "cry it out." Sometimes a fussy baby is crying because he is exhausted and cannot get comfortable. Handling the baby may not be the best thing to do at this time. If you have decided to try letting your baby cry it out, avoid the temptation to run in and check him every few minutes. This only teaches your baby that if he cries long enough he will get someone to hold him.

Remember, however, that at the early stages of an infant's life, he is learning trust. The crying-it-out method should be used carefully and should not be carried to extremes. It is important for you as well as for the baby that you strike a balance between your needs and his. The instructions on the map will help you do this to the benefit of you both.

Try all kinds of things. Make up routines of your own. Go with whatever works. Colic is not permanent. It usually begins at 2 to 3 weeks of age and goes away by 3 to 4 months. Knowing this may be of little comfort at the time you find yourself with a fussy baby, but it is good to know that this fussy period comes to an end.

Sedative medicines should never be given to a baby except on a doctor's instruction. There is almost never a need for these measures. Growing babies need to be active and alert so they can learn about their environment and the people around them.

28. *Growth and Development*

Every baby develops in her own way, at her own pace, influenced by many factors, including her temperament and the environment in which she lives. Researchers over the years have determined the normal range of development by looking at thousands and thousands of babies.

Developmental tasks are often called *milestones*. Sitting, standing, walking, and talking are all major developmental milestones. Doctors speak of children having *normal* or *delayed milestones*. A group of normal babies will achieve each milestone within a certain period of time.

For example, babies normally begin to walk by themselves sometime between 10 and 15 months of age. It is not "better" for a child to walk at 10 months than at 15 months. The child who walks at 15 months may have an older brother and sister who bring everything to her. This child may not feel the need to walk any earlier because she can explore her environment just as easily and comfortably by being waited upon by her older siblings.

Babies will do things when they are ready. Do not try to rush your baby; trust that development will take place in a logical way at a logical pace. For example, a 6-month-old does not have the strength in her bones or muscles to walk, but she may be able to sit by herself.

Development is a process of trial and error. Over a period of weeks to months, progress is easily appreciated. On a day-to-day basis, however, progress is not as easily seen. It is not unusual for a 13-month-old to take a few independent steps one day, and not repeat the feat for several more weeks. Do not worry if your child seems to be developing in this way; it is completely normal.

If you should become concerned about your child's development, discuss the situation with your child's doctor. A routine checkup in the clinic or office is a good time to bring up your concerns. If you feel that you cannot wait until your child's next appointment, call your doctor or clinic during regular office or phone hours.

Growth and Development at Specific Ages

I have listed below, in a general way, the tasks a child usually is able to perform and the ways the child usually acts at specific ages.

AT 1 MONTH OF AGE

Smiles in response to others.

Focuses on objects with her eyes.

Turns her head from side to side.

Cries when she is uncomfortable, wants to be held, is tired or hungry.

Sleeps much of the time.

Eats on the average every 3 to 4½ hours.

Reacts to loud noises.

AT 3 MONTHS OF AGE

Makes cooing noises.

Laughs from time to time.

Lifts her head up high when on her belly.

Rolls over every now and then (she may not do this until 4½ months).

Recognizes her mother.

Follows objects with her eyes and by turning her head.

AT 6 MONTHS OF AGE

Holds her head steady and sits when supported.

Shows signs of displeasure.

Grasps for a toy when it is held near and holds it with surprising strength.

Starts to babble.

Rolls over well.

At 8 Months of Age

Sits without support.

Transfers objects from hand to hand.

Says "mama," or "dada" without meaning (she *may* not do this until 10 months).

Responds to "no."

May act shy with strangers.

Looks briefly for a toy that is taken from her view. (She may not do this until 9 months.)

Feeds herself crackers.

At 10 Months of Age

Sits well.

Crawls on her belly.

Creeps on all fours.

Pulls herself to stand and "cruises" the furniture.

Grasps things by touching her thumb to her index finger.

Waves "bye-bye."

Plays "patty cake," and "peekaboo."

May show preference for one toy over another.

At 12 Months of Age

Walks with support, and may even take a few steps alone. (She may not do this until 13–14 months.)

Says "mama" or "dada" specifically (she *may* not do this until 13 months).

Understands names of objects.

Shows interest in pictures.

Feeds herself finger foods.

May be able to roll a ball to an adult with great pleasure.

May enjoy games of "putting in and taking out."

AT 15 MONTHS OF AGE

Is—or will shortly be—walking alone.

Gives hugs and kisses to her parents.

Imitates adult behavior.

Makes her needs known by pointing.

May become very upset when separated from her parents.

Speaks at least two or three words besides "mama" and "dada" with meaning (she *may* not do this until 20 months).

AT 18 MONTHS OF AGE

Walks up and down the stairs holding on.

Climbs into an adult chair.

Can point to some parts of her body.

Carries out simple commands.

Can remove her clothes.

AT 2 YEARS OF AGE

Runs well.

Walks up and down the stairs by herself.

Begins to engage in fantasy play such as taking care of a teddy bear or "going to the store."

Begins to use pronouns such as *I, you,* and *me.*

May use two- or three-word phrases.

FROM 3 TO 4 YEARS OF AGE

Dresses fully except for tying shoes.

Feeds herself, spilling little.

Plays outside for at least a half hour.

Cares for self at toilet (may need help with wiping).

Copies a circle.

Uses scissors to cut out pictures.

Knows her own sex when asked if she is a boy or girl.

Gives her full name.

Counts up to 10.

Knows many colors.

Asks many questions.

Rides a tricycle or big wheel.

Walks up and down the stairs using each of her feet alternatively.

Hops on one foot.

Skips.

FROM 5 TO 6 YEARS OF AGE

Goes to school unattended or meets the school bus.

Does simple chores at home such as drying the dishes or taking out the garbage.

Dresses completely with no help.

Asks the meaning of words.

Prints a few words.

Copies a triangle or diamond.

Skips well.

Catches a ball.

Knows right from left.

Describes her favorite television show in detail.

Draws a recognizable figure of a person.

Ways to Enhance Your Child's Development

As a parent, you want to give your child the opportunity to reach her full potential in life but you want to avoid being too pushy or compulsive about your child's rate of achievement.

I have outlined below a few things that I feel a parent should consciously try to do with young babies in order to stimulate and challenge them. In general, your interaction with your baby should always be enjoyable, spontaneous, intimate, and warm. These guidelines should not in any way detract from the warmth and spontaneity of your relationship.

Do not worry about buying your baby all kinds of expensive "learning toys." A baby can learn as much about shape, material, texture, and color from playing with the gift wrapping—paper, tissue, box, and ribbon—as from the toy itself. Babies and children are learning machines. They thrive on new experiences and love to explore their environment. It is not the specific activity or toy itself as much as the *process of doing* that enhances development.

Touch and Talk

Young babies are most receptive to touch and sound. They thrive on human interaction. Bathe your baby in language and physical contact. You are your child's guide to the world. Turn chores such as changing diapers and clothes into playtime by doing them with plenty of talking, hugging, tickling, and kissing.

Assume from Birth That Your Baby Understands Everything You Say

Talk to your baby at all times, using the fullest vocabulary possible. *Do not* use baby talk. As they develop, human infants achieve an understanding of language much more rapidly than they learn to talk. As you expose your baby to language, her mind is stimulated and enriched.

Babies and young children are able to learn language at a fantastic rate; their ability is far superior to that of adults. Imagine going to China with your 6-month-old baby, and spending two years there with people who spoke and understood only Chinese. To make matters more difficult, imagine that you had no access to a Chinese-English dictionary. Who do you think would be able to understand Chinese after two years? Your baby!

Talk to your baby about everything and anything. The topic is not important; the exposure to words is what counts. So, as you are changing your 3-month-old, describe the weather, talk about your boss, the upcoming election, the stock market, the NFL, your favorite soap opera, world affairs, or whatever else comes to mind.

READ TO YOUR BABY

Start this as early as you want. Hold your baby on your lap and read picture books to her. Try to do this once a day. In this way books, reading, language, and learning will be pleasant, nonthreatening, and nourishing for your child throughout life.

TURN WORK INTO PLAY

Young children will embrace enthusiastically almost any activity that interests you. For example, make folding laundry into a color-naming game, or shopping into a naming game.

Anna, our 2-year-old, helps us put away the groceries. She tries to name everything we have bought. At times she will put the tuna fish or something similar on the back steps with the laundry detergent, and of course it takes us longer to finish when we let her participate. But what's important is that she is not only building a vocabulary, she is also learning good habits about helping and working.

ASK YOUR CHILD QUESTIONS

This helps stretch your child's intellect and imagination. Because children are unbound by the rigid conventions of society, they will often give surprising answers to what may seem to be the most obvious questions. Thus, you will often be delighted and refreshed by their answers.

DON'T PUSH TOO HARD

There is a danger in over emphasizing your child's development. Be careful not to let your child, especially one of early school-age, feel that she is valued only for her accomplishments. Nourish, but don't force-feed your child expecting a high-performance return. You should let your kids enjoy their childhood without having to perform extraordinary achievements.

29. *Headaches*

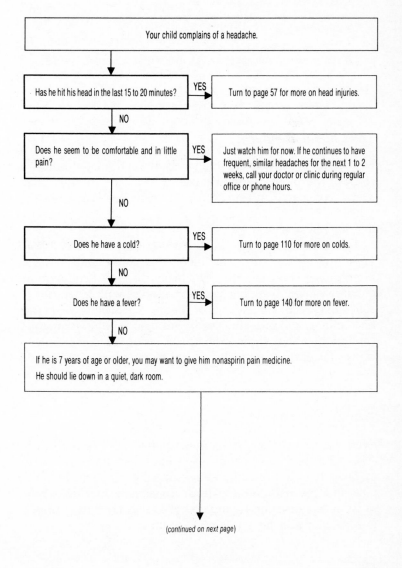

Your child complains of a headache.

Has he hit his head in the last 15 to 20 minutes? — **YES** → Turn to page 57 for more on head injuries.

NO

Does he seem to be comfortable and in little pain? — **YES** → Just watch him for now. If he continues to have frequent, similar headaches for the next 1 to 2 weeks, call your doctor or clinic during regular office or phone hours.

NO

Does he have a cold? — **YES** → Turn to page 110 for more on colds.

NO

Does he have a fever? — **YES** → Turn to page 140 for more on fever.

NO

If he is 7 years of age or older, you may want to give him nonaspirin pain medicine.
He should lie down in a quiet, dark room.

(continued on next page)

(continued from preceding page)

↓

Call your doctor or clinic during regular office or phone hours if:

He has vomited.

He has been awakened from sleep by the headache.

The headache makes him feel sick to his stomach, makes him not want to eat, makes him sensitive to bright light or loud noises.

He is under 8 years of age.

He is not feeling better within the next 24 hours; or he continues to have frequent, similar headaches for the next 1 to 2 weeks.

You have any questions or concerns.

More about Headaches

Headaches are a very common problem with many different causes. The most common types of headache in older children, teenagers, and adults are tension headaches, headaches that accompany congestion from a cold or the flu, and migraine headaches.

Tension headaches occur, but are uncommon in children under the age of 8–10 years. In young children, tension more often causes stomachaches. The headaches most common in children under 10 are headaches that occur with fever, headaches that occur with a cold or the flu, headaches following head injury, and migraine headaches. It is a common misconception that eye strain from poor vision or crossed eyes causes headaches. Actually, eye problems rarely cause headaches.

TENSION HEADACHES

Everyone at one time or another has had this type of headache. Pain from a tension headache is dull and steady. It involves the entire head and is especially worse at the temples and the back of the head. Tension headaches rarely cause severe discomfort, and do not usually force the sufferer to stop whatever he is doing at the time.

Tension headaches are probably caused by prolonged muscle contractions in the neck and scalp triggered by emotional stress or anxiety. Aspirin or nonaspirin pain medicine (acetaminophen) is usually the best treatment for these headaches.

MIGRAINE HEADACHES

Migraine headaches are much less common than tension headaches. They are usually severe headaches, with symptoms that include stomach pain, poor appetite, nausea, and vomiting.

One type of migraine starts with the afflicted person seeing bright flashing spots. This type of migraine is rare in children. Migraines may cause pain on one side of the head, but just as often they involve the entire head. Children and adults who get frequent migraine attacks often want to lie down in a quiet, dark room and go to sleep. The tendency to get migraine headaches is usually inherited; therefore, it is often present in several family members. Children with migraine headaches often have a history of motion sickness as well.

It is sometimes difficult for younger children to express their symptoms clearly, and for this reason migraine headaches may be difficult to detect at an early age.

Migraine headaches are caused by abnormally sensitive blood vessels in the head. These blood vessels change diameter too easily: during a migraine attack they become narrow and then open up too wide. The changes in blood flow stretch the pain-sensitive areas of the head and cause the headache.

Many different things can trigger migraine headaches. Emotional factors are very important. So is diet. Certain foods contain substances called *amines* (pronounced: ah *means*) that can affect blood vessels. These foods include hot dogs and luncheon meats, cheese, chocolate, nuts, and red wine.

There are many different ways to treat migraine headaches. One of the first steps is to try to identify the food triggers and then remove them from the diet. There are many

161

different medicines used to treat migraine headaches, some of which are not safe for children. Some of these medicines are taken all the time in an attempt to prevent headaches. Others are taken just as a headache starts.

In their more severe forms migraine headaches can cause a great deal of suffering. They can be difficult to control. One bright side for migraine sufferers is that the attacks usually cease in late adulthood. Migraine headaches are complicated and chronic. The diagnosis of migraine headaches is best made by a doctor.

30. *Head Lice*

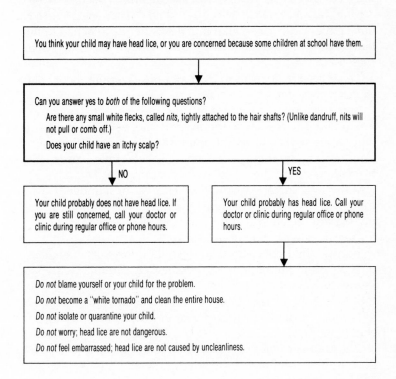

You think your child may have head lice, or you are concerned because some children at school have them.

Can you answer yes to *both* of the following questions?

Are there any small white flecks, called *nits*, tightly attached to the hair shafts? (Unlike dandruff, nits will not pull or comb off.)

Does your child have an itchy scalp?

NO

Your child probably does not have head lice. If you are still concerned, call your doctor or clinic during regular office or phone hours.

YES

Your child probably has head lice. Call your doctor or clinic during regular office or phone hours.

Do not blame yourself or your child for the problem.

Do not become a "white tornado" and clean the entire house.

Do not isolate or quarantine your child.

Do not worry; head lice are not dangerous.

Do not feel embarrassed; head lice are not caused by uncleanliness.

More about Head Lice

Head lice are a worldwide problem. School-age children are most commonly affected, but the problem can occur at any age. In fact, this country is experiencing a head-lice epidemic among school-age children.

Head lice are tiny parasites that live on the skin surface and hair of humans. Being parasites, they cannot survive for more than a few days separated from a human body. Head lice are passed on by close contact with an infested person or by close contact with the personal belongings of an infested person, such as a comb or bedclothes.

Head lice usually cause intense itching, which is worse during the night. Head lice eggs, called *nits,* are visible to the naked eye. Look for small white flecks tightly attached to the hair shafts. Unlike dandruff, they cannot be combed or pulled off.

Head lice are not caused by poor housekeeping, poor child care, or poor personal habits.

Head lice do not carry infection and are not dangerous. Treatment is with a prescription shampoo, usually used twice within one week's time. It is important to rinse off the shampoo thoroughly after use. Clothes, sheets, pillowcases, and blankets used by the infested child during the two days before the first shampoo should be cleaned or laundered. Use the hot cycle of your washing machine. Dry cleaning or simply storing the clothes and bedclothes in a closed plastic bag for ten days will also kill head lice.

If your child contracts head lice, all household members, including the adults, should be checked carefully. Anyone found to have head lice should be treated as well. If the infested child shares a bed with someone, her bedmate should be treated even if you cannot find any nits in the child's hair.

A school-age child can easily become reinfested with head lice through continued exposure to infested classmates.

The medical term for head lice infestation is *pediculosis* (pronounced: pih dick yuh *low* suss).

31. *Newborn Babies*

Newborn babies are wonderful beings. To the new parents they may also seem unusual, different, and strange. I will discuss on the following pages many features of newborn babies that parents often wonder about. I have divided the discussion into three major categories covering newborn appearance, newborn behavior, and caring for newborn babies.

What Newborn Babies Look Like

Body hair.   Newborn babies may be covered entirely with soft, fine hair which can be of any color. This hair, whose medical name is *lanugo* (pronounced luh *nyoo* go), soon falls off.

Birthmarks.   Newborn babies usually have red, blotchy birthmarks on the back of the neck. This "stork bite," as it is often called, fades with time. Black and Asian babies have birthmarks that look like inkblots on their upper bottoms. These too fade with time.

Breathing.   Newborn babies breathe at a rapid rate, normally at 30 to 40 breaths a minute. This can increase to 60 breaths a minute with excitement. The newborn breathes almost entirely through his nose.

Breasts.   The breasts of newborn babies of both sexes will be somewhat enlarged. Occasionally the nipples produce tiny amounts of milk. These effects are caused by the mother's hormones stimulating the unborn baby's breast tissues. This is a temporary effect which disappears soon after birth.

Bulges around belly buttons. Newborn babies, especially black babies, may have a large bulge in the belly-button region. The bulge gets bigger when the baby cries. It can be quite large, up to a couple of inches in diameter and height. This bulge is a called an *umbilical hernia*. It gradually disappears during the first several years of life. Umbilical hernias are not dangerous and rarely ever require treatment.

Bumps and bruises. During birth your baby may become bruised and bumped. His head may be very irregular, looking something like a football. This is because the bones of the scalp are able to slide around, allowing the head to pass through the birth canal. Bruising and swelling of the scalp also may occur. Forcep marks are red, curved bruises that mark the face. These are not permanent problems. Usually they resolve during the first several weeks of life.

Cradle cap. A week or two after birth, babies commonly develop thick, yellow, greasy patches on the scalp; the patches look something like small potato chips. This condition, called *cradle cap*, is not dangerous. If the scaling becomes thick and adherent, you can apply warmed mineral oil to the scalp before you shampoo the baby's hair.

Eyes. Newborn babies will open their eyes for brief periods of time. They are sensitive to bright lights. A good way to get a newborn to open his eyes is to have him suck on your finger or drink from a bottle. By 2 to 4 weeks of age, babies will start looking around and focusing on objects. Newborns may have a fluid discharge from the eyes for several days. This is usually due to the disinfectant placed in the eyes just after birth.

Genitals. Newborn female babies may have swollen vaginal folds. Often there is a small amount of bleeding or white fluid discharge from the vagina as well. These effects are caused by the mother's hormones, which stimulate the vagina in the womb. They will disappear in a very short time. Male babies often have fluid in the testicular sac. This is not dangerous, and the fluid will slowly disappear over several weeks. If you are concerned that your child may have a hernia, discuss the matter with your doctor.

Length. Babies are usually between 17 and 21 inches long at birth.

Jaundice. Newborn babies at 1 to 3 days of age will turn yellow in varying degrees. This is termed *jaundice*. The yellow skin color is completely normal and is expected in newborn babies. Jaundice in newborns is caused by immature red blood cells breaking down to form bilirubin. The bilirubin is then deposited in the skin. The yellow color that forms around black-and-blue marks is caused by a similar process. Hospitals often put more heavily jaundiced babies under blue lights to hasten the breakdown of bilirubin and prevent the rare situation of bilirubin reaching too high a level. Breast-fed babies will stay jaundiced longer.

Meconium. For the first several days of life, babies' bowels are filled with a very thick and sticky dark green substance called *meconium* (pronounced: mih *koh* knee um), which they discharge during bowel movements. At times a baby will have a meconium bowel movement in the birth canal during delivery. This occasionally causes breathing problems.

Soft spots on the head. Newborns have two soft spots under the scalp: one above the forehead, and one small one at the back of the head. These soft spots allow for the hard, bony skull to be safely compressed and molded during passage through the birth canal. It is all right to gently touch and wash these areas. It is normal to feel a pulse through the soft spots. The soft spot in back is sometimes already closed by birth; otherwise, it usually closes within 2 to 4 months after birth. The soft spot in front closes completely within 10 to 18 months. The medical term for these soft spots is *fontanel* (pronounced: font un *el*).

Temperature. The normal body temperature of a newborn baby is between 98° and 100° Fahrenheit (36.7° to 37.8° Celsius).

Thrush. Soon after birth, a newborn baby may develop a yeast infection of the mouth called *thrush*. This appears as white patches on the inside of the mouth, usually on the tongue and inside of the cheeks. The white patches look like formula or breast milk, but unlike food, the patches cannot be wiped away. Thrush is not dangerous; it can make a baby uncomfortable though. Thrush is treated with a prescription medicine that is squirted into the mouth three or four times a day for 7 to 10 days. Call your doctor or clinic during regular office or phone hours if you think your baby may have thrush.

Umbilical cord. The umbilical cord will fall off when your baby is 1 to 2 weeks of age. The blue color of the cord is due to an antiseptic dye that is painted on the cord soon after delivery. It is best to clean the cord with rubbing alcohol three or four times a day. Use a cotton ball or cotton swab to apply the alcohol. Do not cover the umbilical cord with a bandage or tape; let it dry in the open air. Do not try to pull off the cord.

Weight. Full-term babies usually weigh between 4½ and 8½ pounds. A newborn baby will loose up to 10 percent of his body weight during the first 7 to 10 days of life. Babies are born with an excess amount of body water which protects them against dehydration during the first few days of life. Babies will double their birth weight within 5 or 6 months after birth, and triple their birth weight within 10 to 12 months.

How Newborn Babies Behave

Newborn babies eat, sleep, and cry when they are uncomfortable. It is not unusual for a newborn to sleep between 12 and

20 hours a day. They sleep so much because their energy is almost entirely consumed by growing; they have very little energy for anything else.

Do not be fooled by your newborn baby's limited number of activities. He is very sensitive to the outside world, with touch and hearing being his strongest senses. Babies react very well to a gentle voice, touch, caress, or kiss. Newborns love to be cuddled and held tightly. This is why swaddling works so nicely. Babies respond positively to being moved about. Rocking is usually most comforting to newborns.

Your baby will learn and develop at a rapid pace. By 1 month of age, he will focus on objects, smile responsively to faces, and react with a start to loud noises. Turn to Chapter 28, "Growth and Development," for more details.

Care of Newborn Babies

While newborn babies require special care and handling, they should not be handled as if they might break suddenly. Careful handling can be taken to unnecessary extremes. New parents are often understandably concerned that their baby will be easily injured even by gentle handling. Babies are not like fine pieces of delicate crystal, however. They are really fairly rugged. So don't be afraid to hug and squeeze your new baby.

Below are some specific details concerning the care of newborn babies.

Bathing.   Newborn babies can be sponge-bathed first when they are 2 days old. Do not fully immerse a newborn in a tub of water until the umbilical cord has fallen off. To bathe your baby, use water that is comfortably warm to your touch.

Carrying and holding.   For the first several weeks of life a baby needs to have his head supported when he is not lying down.

Circumcision.   There is no medical reason for performing a circumcision. Recent research has established that there are *no* health benefits from this procedure, either to males or their female partners. Circumcision has a very low but real complication rate. It has become standard practice in the United States that probably should be discontinued except among those who wish to have the procedure performed for religious reasons. If your baby is circumcised, his penis should be coated with petroleum jelly with every other diaper change until the redness subsides; this usually takes a few days.

Dressing.   Newborn babies can be taken outside safely at 2 to 3 days of age—unless the weather is severe. Newborn babies are probably greatly overdressed in general. Adequate dress for newborns includes a diaper and undershirt; sleeper, sleep bag, or jumper; and a light crib blanket. When taking your baby outside, make sure his head, hands, and feet are well covered. Use yourself as a barometer. If you feel chilly and need a sweater, put one on your baby. If you become hot, take off your own sweater and the baby's as well.

Feeding.   Babies eat very little the first day of life. Those on formula may take a half ounce of sugar water, and then formula every three to four hours. Breast-fed babies stay at the breast for up to five minutes, with the same frequency. Your baby's appetite will increase slowly. By the time your baby is 2 weeks old, his feeding routine is usually 2 to 4 ounces (or 5 to 15 minutes on the breast) every 2½ to 4 hours. To learn more, turn to Chapter 25, "Feeding Babies and Young Children."

Pacifiers.   It is fine to use pacifiers. They are not habit-forming (how many 25-year-olds have you seen using them?) and harmless to the baby. They safely and often quickly calm, soothe, quiet, and comfort babies.

Room temperature.   Your baby's room should be kept at 70° to 72° Fahrenheit (21.1° to 22.2° Celsius) for the first few weeks. Once your baby is 1 month old, it is fine to let the temperature drop at night to between 65° and 68° Fahrenheit (18.3° and 20° Celsius). Avoid the temptation to overheat your baby's room.

Traveling.   Whenever you travel with your baby place him securely in an infant car-safety seat. *Take your baby home from the hospital in a car-safety seat.* These seats are discussed in detail in Chapter 43, "Prevention of Accidents."

Sleeping.   A newborn baby should be placed on his belly or side when put down to sleep. A pillow or blanket roll works well to keep a baby on his side. Avoid putting a young baby down to sleep on his back. A baby can spit up food even an hour or two after eating, and if this should occur while a young baby is on his back, breathing problems could occur. This becomes much less of a concern by 6 months of age, when babies have stopped spitting up their food to a great extent. After 6 months of age, babies can be put down to sleep in any position.

32. *Nosebleeds*

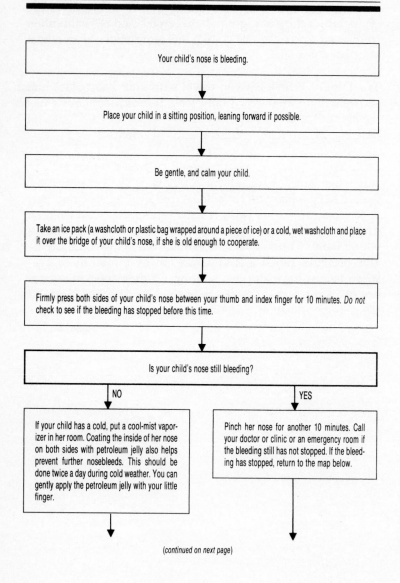

Your child's nose is bleeding.

↓

Place your child in a sitting position, leaning forward if possible.

↓

Be gentle, and calm your child.

↓

Take an ice pack (a washcloth or plastic bag wrapped around a piece of ice) or a cold, wet washcloth and place it over the bridge of your child's nose, if she is old enough to cooperate.

↓

Firmly press both sides of your child's nose between your thumb and index finger for 10 minutes. *Do not* check to see if the bleeding has stopped before this time.

↓

Is your child's nose still bleeding?

NO

If your child has a cold, put a cool-mist vaporizer in her room. Coating the inside of her nose on both sides with petroleum jelly also helps prevent further nosebleeds. This should be done twice a day during cold weather. You can gently apply the petroleum jelly with your little finger.

YES

Pinch her nose for another 10 minutes. Call your doctor or clinic or an emergency room if the bleeding still has not stopped. If the bleeding has stopped, return to the map below.

(continued on next page)

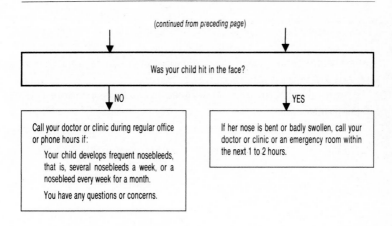

(continued from preceding page)

Was your child hit in the face?

NO

Call your doctor or clinic during regular office or phone hours if:

Your child develops frequent nosebleeds, that is, several nosebleeds a week, or a nosebleed every week for a month.

You have any questions or concerns.

YES

If her nose is bent or badly swollen, call your doctor or clinic or an emergency room within the next 1 to 2 hours.

More about Nosebleeds

Nosebleeds are usually caused by injury from nose picking or sneezing associated with colds or allergies. Indoor heating during the winter can dry out and crack the lining of the nose.

Of course, a blow to the nose can also cause it to bleed. It is important to remember that a broken nose does not always bleed. Conversely, an injured nose that is bleeding is not necessarily broken. As outlined on the map, a broken nose should be suspected following trauma if it appears to be bent or badly swollen.

A bleeding child can be a very frightening sight for parents. It only takes a tablespoon of blood to cover an entire shirt front. Most nosebleeds, however, cause only a small amount of blood loss.

Frequent nosebleeds, especially from the same side of the nose, can be a problem. They are often caused by a small sore in the lining of the nose that never completely heals. This is called a *bleeding point*. To stop the nosebleeds, it may be necessary to have a doctor form a scar over the bleeding point.

This is done with a small rod that passes a tiny amount of electrical current to the bleeding point. This procedure is called *cauterization* (pronounced: caught uh ruh *zay* shun); it is usually quite safe and is not very painful.

The medical term for a nosebleed is *epistaxis* (pronounced: epp eh *stack* suss).

33. *Pinkeye and Sties*

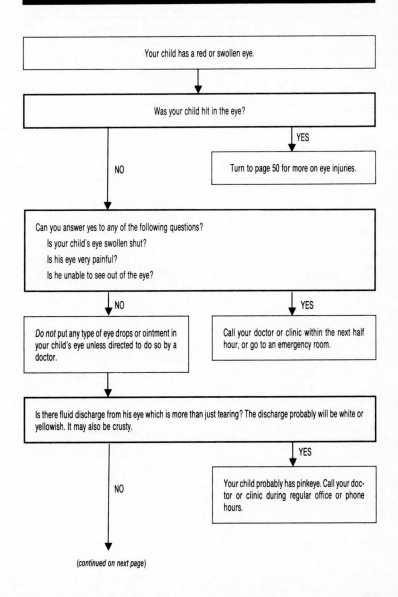

Your child has a red or swollen eye.

↓

Was your child hit in the eye?

YES → Turn to page 50 for more on eye injuries.

NO ↓

Can you answer yes to *any* of the following questions?
  Is your child's eye swollen shut?
  Is his eye very painful?
  Is he unable to see out of the eye?

NO ↓

Do not put any type of eye drops or ointment in your child's eye unless directed to do so by a doctor.

YES ↓

Call your doctor or clinic within the next half hour, or go to an emergency room.

↓

Is there fluid discharge from his eye which is more than just tearing? The discharge probably will be white or yellowish. It may also be crusty.

YES ↓

Your child probably has pinkeye. Call your doctor or clinic during regular office or phone hours.

NO ↓

(continued on next page)

(continued from preceding page)

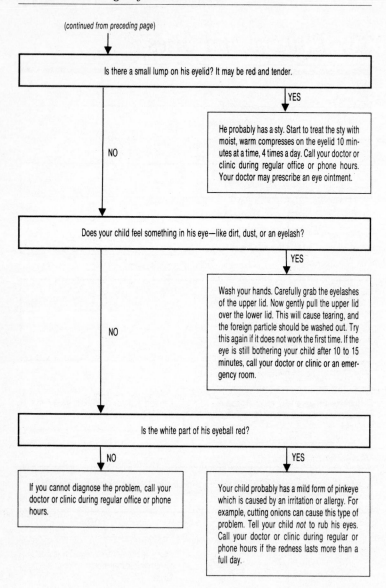

Is there a small lump on his eyelid? It may be red and tender.

YES

He probably has a sty. Start to treat the sty with moist, warm compresses on the eyelid 10 minutes at a time, 4 times a day. Call your doctor or clinic during regular office or phone hours. Your doctor may prescribe an eye ointment.

NO

Does your child feel something in his eye—like dirt, dust, or an eyelash?

YES

Wash your hands. Carefully grab the eyelashes of the upper lid. Now gently pull the upper lid over the lower lid. This will cause tearing, and the foreign particle should be washed out. Try this again if it does not work the first time. If the eye is still bothering your child after 10 to 15 minutes, call your doctor or clinic or an emergency room.

NO

Is the white part of his eyeball red?

NO

If you cannot diagnose the problem, call your doctor or clinic during regular office or phone hours.

YES

Your child probably has a mild form of pinkeye which is caused by an irritation or allergy. For example, cutting onions can cause this type of problem. Tell your child *not* to rub his eyes. Call your doctor or clinic during regular or phone hours if the redness lasts more than a full day.

More about Pinkeye and Sties

PINKEYE

Pinkeye is caused by irritation of the eye; the usual source of the irritation is an infection or allergy. The medical term for pinkeye is *conjunctivitis* (pronounced: con junk tuh *vite* us).

Pinkeye caused by infections can be very contagious. The child tends to rub his eyes, which just irritates them more and usually spreads the infection from one eye to the other. Conjunctivitis often develops when a child has a cold.

It's a good idea to have a child use a separate washcloth and towel while he has conjunctivitis. He should not go into a swimming pool until his conjunctivitis has been gone for three or four days. This prevents people who use the pool from catching your child's conjunctivitis.

Pinkeye caused by infections is best treated by prescription antibiotic eye ointment. Most doctors prescribe that the ointment be put in *both* eyes. It is usually used for a week to 10 days. If the eye stays red or if the discharge returns, call your doctor.

Pinkeye caused by allergies is not contagious. This type of conjunctivitis usually occurs in children who have hay fever. It is often treated with an antihistamine (a type of anti-allergy medicine) taken by mouth. Often an eye ointment or drop medication is also necessary.

Never give your child any type of medicine for eye problems unless directed to do so by a doctor.

STIES

A sty is actually a pimple of the eyelid. It is caused by an infection in a lubricating gland in the eyelid. Treat a sty with moist, warm compresses, which bring the pimple to a head. Antibiotic eye drops are often prescribed as well. The medical term for sty is *hordeolum* (pronounced: hor *de* o lum).

34. *Pinworms*

You think your child may have pinworms, or you are concerned because some children at school have them.

Can you answer yes to *most* of the following questions?

Does your child keep scratching herself around the anus (the *anus* is where bowel movements leave the body), or if your child is a girl, around the vaginal area?

Does her scratching increase at night?

Is she in a preschool program or elementary school?

Is it between October and late spring?

NO

Your child probably does not have pinworms. If you are still concerned, call your doctor or clinic during regular office or phone hours.

YES

Your child may have pinworms. Call your doctor or clinic during regular office or phone hours. Do not worry: pinworm infections are a nuisance, but they are *not dangerous*. The only way to treat the itching from pinworms is with a prescription medicine from your doctor.

If your child should wake up in the middle of the night with itching, check to see if you can find any pinworms. They are small, white-yellow worms about ¼ to ⅓ of an inch long. If you see any worms, take some tape and pick up a few worms with the sticky side of the tape. Put them in a jar of rubbing alcohol and bring it with you to the doctor's office.

(continued on next page)

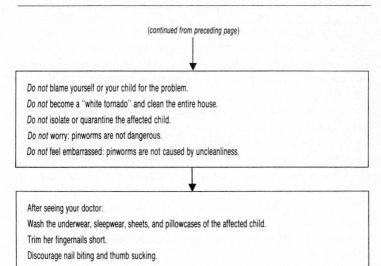

(continued from preceding page)

Do not blame yourself or your child for the problem.

Do not become a "white tornado" and clean the entire house.

Do not isolate or quarantine the affected child.

Do not worry: pinworms are not dangerous.

Do not feel embarrassed: pinworms are not caused by uncleanliness.

After seeing your doctor:

Wash the underwear, sleepwear, sheets, and pillowcases of the affected child.

Trim her fingernails short.

Discourage nail biting and thumb sucking.

More about Pinworms

Pinworms are small worms that can infect people. They are yellow-white in color and a quarter to a third of an inch long. They can be seen with the naked eye.

Pinworms are found all over the world. They are more common in temperate climates like that of the United States. Pinworm infections usually occur between October and late spring.

Pinworm infections occur in people of all ages but most commonly in young children in preschool programs and elementary school. Children at these ages play and sleep close together, which promotes the spread of the worms. Pinworm infections are *not* caused by poor housekeeping, poor child care, or poor personal habits.

Adult pinworms live in the lower end of the intestines, called the *colon*. A pregnant female pinworm leaves the colon of the infected person through the anus and deposits eggs in the skin around the anus. This usually happens at night, and the presence of the eggs causes nighttime itching and scratching. Sometimes the pregnant pinworm deposits its eggs in the outside folds of the infected child's vagina. This is why girls with pinworm infections will often complain of vaginal itching. Pinworm eggs are too small to be seen with the naked eye.

Once the eggs are deposited on the skin, they stick to fingernails if the infected person scratches the anal area. The eggs can be passed back into the person's own digestive system if she puts her hands in her mouth. The eggs travel to the intestines and develop into adult pinworms. A person can pick up the eggs through close contact with an infected person or through the handling of an infected person's underwear or bedclothes that contain the eggs.

Pinworm infections do not cause abdominal pain or any other type of medical problem. In fact, they cause only the types of itching and scratching described above. Pinworm infections are not in any way dangerous or life-threatening.

Pinworm infections are safely, easily, and effectively treated with a prescription medicine which is taken by mouth. The medicine is taken in a single dose and is repeated in two or three weeks. The medicine can be taken as either a chewable tablet or as a liquid. It is usually best to treat *all* members of the family, even if others do not have symptoms. The only exception would be a pregnant woman. The medicine may cause an upset stomach for a brief time, and the liquid can occasionally cause mild drowsiness.

Your doctor may ask you to help him or her make the diagnosis by using the "Scotch tape test" to detect pinworm eggs. It is performed as follows: Upon a child's first awakening and before going to the bathroom, an adult takes a piece of clear Scotch tape and places the sticky side against the child's bottom just next to the anus. This is repeated a couple of times in different places around the anus. Then the tape is placed on a glass microscope slide and brought to the doctor's office. (Your doctor will provide the slide.)

Do not go wild trying to fumigate your entire house if someone in the family is found to have pinworms. A thorough washing of the infected child's underwear, sleepwear, sheets, and pillowcases is all that is required. Be careful not to make your child feel she is to blame for getting the infection. Do not isolate the child or make her feel "dirty" or contagious.

Pinworm infections can recur easily, as children from different families pass the infection back and forth. Repeated infections are treated in the same way as the first infection.

35. *Rashes*

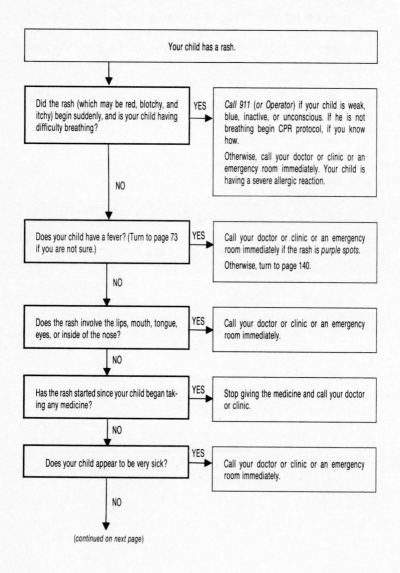

Your child has a rash.

Did the rash (which may be red, blotchy, and itchy) begin suddenly, and is your child having difficulty breathing?

YES → *Call 911 (or Operator)* if your child is weak, blue, inactive, or unconscious. If he is not breathing begin CPR protocol, if you know how.

Otherwise, call your doctor or clinic or an emergency room immediately. Your child is having a severe allergic reaction.

NO ↓

Does your child have a fever? (Turn to page 73 if you are not sure.)

YES → Call your doctor or clinic or an emergency room immediately if the rash is *purple spots*.

Otherwise, turn to page 140.

NO ↓

Does the rash involve the lips, mouth, tongue, eyes, or inside of the nose?

YES → Call your doctor or clinic or an emergency room immediately.

NO ↓

Has the rash started since your child began taking any medicine?

YES → Stop giving the medicine and call your doctor or clinic.

NO ↓

Does your child appear to be very sick?

YES → Call your doctor or clinic or an emergency room immediately.

NO ↓

(continued on next page)

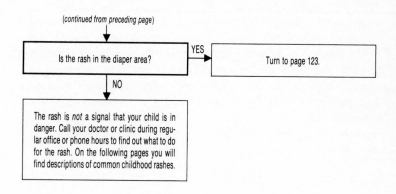

(continued from preceding page)

Is the rash in the diaper area? — **YES** → Turn to page 123.

NO

The rash is *not* a signal that your child is in danger. Call your doctor or clinic during regular office or phone hours to find out what to do for the rash. On the following pages you will find descriptions of common childhood rashes.

More about Rashes

Children frequently get rashes. One reason is that their skin is more delicate than the skin of adults. Most rashes are not dangerous. The map at the beginning of this chapter will help you decide how to deal with your child's rash.

Skin rashes have many causes. A rash can be caused by the direct infection of the skin by a germ (as in chicken pox or athlete's foot), by the dilation of small blood vessels (as in hives), by an allergic reaction (as in a drug rash), or by direct irritation of the skin (as in contact dermatitis). Rashes vary in their duration; they can last several minutes or many months.

Listed below are common rashes occurring in childhood. Many of these rashes also affect adults. The list is not given as an aid in diagnosing your child's rash. It is intended to help you understand more about your child's rash once it has been diagnosed by a doctor.

ATHLETE'S FOOT

Athlete's foot is an itchy rash on the soles of the feet and between the toes. It is caused by a fungus germ; it is actually ringworm of the feet. Athlete's foot occurs all over the world and affects primarily people who wear shoes. It is picked up in damp places such as locker rooms and shower rooms.

Athlete's foot is treated with fungus-killing medicine. There are prescription and nonprescription medicines for athlete's foot in cream and powder form. The medicine is placed directly on the rash. Treatment and prevention measures include keeping the feet clean, cool, dry, and well aerated. Drying between the toes after bathing or swimming is also recommended. Your doctor may recommend a plain drying powder to be used as well in between applications of the medicine. Treatment may take several months.

Athlete's foot is not dangerous, and there is no need to isolate the affected person. This rash rarely occurs before the teenage years. The medical term for athlete's foot is *tinea pedis* (pronounced: *tin* ee uh   *ped* iss).

CHICKEN POX

Chicken pox is caused by a viral infection that affects the entire body. It usually occurs in 5- to 10-year-olds. Almost everyone gets chicken pox before reaching adulthood; an adult who assumes he or she never had chicken pox probably in fact had a mild case during childhood. You can have chicken pox only once.

The rash can appear suddenly without warning, or it may be preceded by several days of mild fever and a runny nose. The rash usually starts on the face and moves downward, eventually covering the entire body. The rash appears first as small, flat red dots which change into small bumps and then into clear pimples which finally break and crust over. The rash breaks out in "crops" of lesions over four to five days. At any one time, parts of the rash will just be beginning as flat dots and other parts already will have crusted. A child may be covered with a few or several hundred different spots at the height of the rash. Chicken pox usually lasts seven to ten days.

Chicken pox is extremely contagious. An affected child is contagious for one or two days before the rash appears and until there are no new spots and the entire rash has reached the crusted stage. Chicken pox is spread by direct contact or coughing. A child can come down with this infection ten days to three weeks after being exposed to it. Chicken pox commonly runs through kindergarten and elementary schools during the late winter and early spring.

There is no treatment for chicken pox except to take care of the symptoms such as fever and itching. Despite active research on a vaccine, there is presently no vaccine available for preventing chicken pox. Antibiotics have no effect on this disease.

A child with chicken pox should be kept home from school for at least seven days from the time the rash starts. Your child should not return to school until all the rash has reached the crusted stage. (It may take several weeks for the crusty rash to disappear). You do not have to isolate your sick child from the rest of the family, since exposure has already occurred by the time the rash has developed.

Children with chicken pox usually do well and recover fully. They usually do not act very ill; however, some children may be particularly uncomfortable and irritable for several days. Watch your child for vomiting or unusual hostility, irritability, and other bizzare behavior during the recovery phase. Let your doctor know immediately if any vomiting develops. This may be the first sign of Reye's syndrome (see Chapter 36). Do not give your child aspirin while he has chicken pox or for two weeks afterward; it is fine to give nonaspirin fever medicine (acetaminophen). Recent research has linked Reye's syndrome with the use of aspirin with children who have had the flu or chicken pox.

The skin heals without scarring provided the child does not scratch the crusted pimples. (As a child, I frequently scratched one chicken pock on my forehead, and to this day I have a small scar.) Chicken pox is very itchy. Keep your child's fingernails short. You can put calamine or similar lotion on the rash. Your child will look "painted" with dots from head to toe. A colloidal oatmeal bath, such as Aveeno®, can be quite soothing. If the itching becomes severe, your doctor can prescribe anti-itching medicine.

If you have a house full of small children, be prepared: probably all of them will come down with chicken pox, one after the other, once it has entered your house.

The medical name for chicken pox is *varicella* (pronounced: vare uh *sell* uh).

CONTACT DERMATITIS

Contact dermatitis is a red, itchy, scaly rash. It is caused by direct skin contact with substances to which certain individuals are sensitive. The nickel found in watches is a very common cause of contact dermatitis. Fur, leather, and fabric dyes can cause this rash. Poison ivy, poison oak, and poison sumac are all forms of contact dermatitis. The rash only occurs where direct contact has been made.

Contact dermatitis is treated by removing the offending agent. Sometimes an anti-itching cream such as hydrocortisone is prescribed. But even medicines applied to sensitized skin can cause contact dermatitis, so medicines are kept to a minimum when treating this type of rash. Contact dermatitis is not contagious.

DRUG RASHES

Medicines taken by any route can cause rashes. Medicines are foreign substances, and as such they can trigger allergic reactions. The rashes take many forms, the most common of which are hives or a fine, red, bumpy, itchy rash. As directed in the map, if your child develops a rash after starting a medicine, stop giving the medicine and call your doctor or clinic. Drug rashes are not contagious.

ECZEMA

Eczema has been called "an itch that rashes." Its cause is not known, but it happens to people who have sensitive skin. The itching can be triggered by many different things, including contact with clothing, temperature changes, sweating, dryness, contact with rough materials, and certain detergents.

Eczema can begin at any age. It usually lasts a long time; it may even last a lifetime. In infants the rash occurs mostly on the face and trunk. In older individuals the rash tends to concentrate behind the neck, behind the knees, and on the front of the elbows.

Treatment of eczema begins with keeping the skin moist. Try to keep baths to a minimum. Use nonirritating soaps such as Dove®, Neutrogena®, Basis®, or Lowila®. Rinse off the soap thoroughly before your child leaves the tub. Pat the skin dry as soon as your child gets out of the tub. Do not let the skin air-dry after a bath, since this dries out the skin.

Use a bland cream such as Eucerin® or mineral oil to keep the skin moist; apply it three times a day. You may want to try Alpha-Keri® or Aveeno® added to the water halfway through the bath (this leaves an oily film on the tub, though). Keep your child's fingernails short. Avoid any laundry detergents that seem to make the rash worse. Wool and other materials should be avoided if they make itching worse.

If itching becomes more severe, your doctor may suggest hydrocortisone or some other type of cream. Severe itching can also be treated with anti-itching medicines (antihistamines) taken by mouth; they can make your child sleepy, however. Remember that eczema is not contagious.

HIVES

Hives are large, red, blotchy, flat bumps that can be very itchy. They usually begin suddenly and last for several hours at a time. Hives are caused by dilation of blood vessels which produces patches of skin swelling. Hives change in appearance rapidly and can appear to "move" over the skin.

There are a great many possible triggering agents for hives, including cold weather; cold water; certain medicines; and certain foods, especially fish, nuts, peanuts, and eggs. It is often difficult to determine just what triggered the appearance of hives in a specific child.

The treatment of hives includes avoidance of the triggering agents when they can be determined. Your doctor may prescribe an anti-itching medicine, which is often given at night because of its tendency to cause sleepiness.

Hives by themselves are not dangerous. They can be accompanied by breathing problems, however, due to swelling of the upper breathing passages. This can be a very dangerous situation. As directed on the map, you should obtain medical help *immediately* if any breathing problem occurs with hives. A child who has had an attack of hives with associated breathing problems may have to carry a preloaded syringe containing *epinephrine* (pronounced: epp eh *neff* rin) and be taught how to give himself an injection in an emergency.

Any one episode of hives rarely lasts longer than two weeks. However, repeated episodes can occur over months to years.

The medical term for hives is *urticaria* (pronounced: urt uh *care* ee uh). Hives are not contagious.

IMPETIGO

Impetigo appears as multiple small, irregular, red patches which have a honey-colored crust. Impetigo most commonly occurs on the face, especially around the mouth and nostrils, but may also occur on the arms and legs. Impetigo either has no symptoms or is only mildly itchy.

Impetigo commonly follows a minor skin injury, insect bite, or sting. Infants may get impetigo because frequent drooling can make the skin around the mouth irritated and prone to infection. Impetigo is *not* usually caused by poor hygiene. Do not blame yourself or your child if impetigo occurs.

Impetigo is caused by bacteria. An antibiotic is given orally for 7 to 10 days. Older children can at times be treated with an antibiotic ointment which is applied to the rash. It is a good idea to cut fingernails short until the impetigo clears. This will prevent spread to other parts of the body.

Impetigo is mildly contagious—close contact with an infected person is usually required. It is not necessary to isolate a child with impetigo; however, washcloths and towels should not be shared with other family members until the rash clears.

MEASLES AND GERMAN MEASLES

These illnesses are both rare in the United States due to our program of immunization. The measles, mumps, and rubella (MMR) vaccine (see Chapter 44, "Immunizations") protects against both these illnesses as well as against mumps. What people call *the measles* is usually a viral rash (see description at the end of this section).

RINGWORM

Ringworm is a round, itchy rash with a red-edged ring; it can occur anywhere on the body. The rash most often consists of one or two patches; usually the patches are the size of a quarter or silver dollar, but they can be even larger.

Ringworm is *not* caused by a worm infection. It is caused by a fungus infection. One catches ringworm by direct contact with an infected person or animal, usually a cat. It is not necessary to isolate a child who has ringworm from other children. Ringworm is not dangerous.

Ringworm of the scalp is treated with medicine which is taken by mouth. Ringworm of the rest of the body usually is treated with an ointment applied directly to the rash. Treatment usually takes several weeks.

The medical term for ringworm of the scalp is *tinea capitis* (pronounced: *tin* ee uh   *cap* it iss), and ringworm of the body is called *tinea corporis* (pronounced: *tin* ee uh   *cor* por us). Ringworm of the feet is athlete's foot (see above).

ROSEOLA

Roseola is a type of viral rash (see below). It occurs in infants shortly after a two- or three-day fever has broken. Infants with roseola do not act very sick and the condition is not dangerous, however, it is slightly contagious. There is no treatment required for an infant who has roseola.

SCABIES

Scabies is a red rash that is extremely itchy. It may begin between the fingers and then spread to other parts of the body. The scabies rash is caused by a type of parasite called a *mite*. Mites are insects that look something like spiders; they are too small to be seen with the naked eye, however. Mites do *not* nest in the hair.

The itching is caused by mites burrowing in the skin, and it is often worse at night. Scabies is treated by a prescription lotion which is placed on the entire body from the neck down. The lotion is left on for several hours and then washed off. Two or three treatments are usually necessary.

Scabies is passed on by close contact with infected individuals. The rash is not dangerous, and it is not necessary to isolate a child who has scabies. However, it is important to make sure that *all family members,* not just the infected child or adult, are treated—even if they do not have symptoms of scabies. The infected individual's clothing, sheets, pillowcases, and blankets should be washed thoroughly.

SEBORRHEA

Seborrhea (pronounced: seb uh *ree* uh) is an itchy, scaly rash. It is not dangerous, though it can last a lifetime. Dandruff is seborrhea of the scalp (called *cradle cap* in infants; see Chapter 31, "Newborn Babies"). Seborrhea often occurs in skin folds. This rash is treated with prescription and nonprescription ointments such as hydrocortisone. It is not contagious.

VIRAL RASHES

A cold, the flu, or fever alone in children is often accompanied by a rash. These ailments are caused by germs called *viruses*. The rashes that accompany them are usually fine red bumps that are mildly itchy. The rashes themselves are not dangerous and do not require any treatment.

36. *Reye's Syndrome*

Reye's (pronounced: rise) syndrome is a rare but dangerous illness that can follow the flu or chicken pox.

Chicken pox is discussed on page 184. The flu is an illness caused by a type of germ called a *virus*. It almost always occurs during winter months, often in epidemics. The flu begins rapidly with hacking cough, followed by high fever, chills, headache, muscle aches, discomfort, and lack of energy. *Flu* is another term for influenza.

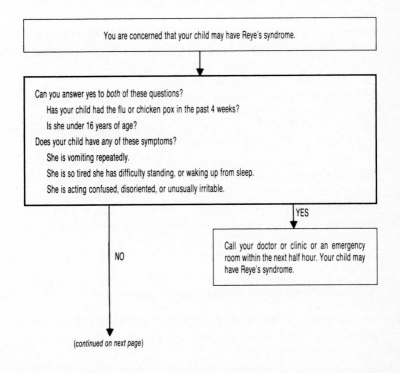

You are concerned that your child may have Reye's syndrome.

Can you answer yes to *both* of these questions?

    Has your child had the flu or chicken pox in the past 4 weeks?

    Is she under 16 years of age?

Does your child have *any* of these symptoms?

    She is vomiting repeatedly.

    She is so tired she has difficulty standing, or waking up from sleep.

    She is acting confused, disoriented, or unusually irritable.

YES

Call your doctor or clinic or an emergency room within the next half hour. Your child may have Reye's syndrome.

NO

(continued on next page)

(continued from preceding page)

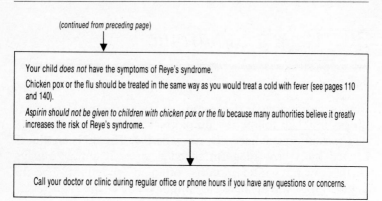

Your child *does not* have the symptoms of Reye's syndrome.

Chicken pox or the flu should be treated in the same way as you would treat a cold with fever (see pages 110 and 140).

Aspirin should not be given to children with chicken pox or the flu because many authorities believe it greatly increases the risk of Reye's syndrome.

Call your doctor or clinic during regular office or phone hours if you have any questions or concerns.

More about Reye's Syndrome

Reye's syndrome is an illness of unknown cause. It occurs in children who are recovering from the flu or chicken pox. Reye's syndrome is *not* caused by the flu or chicken pox itself, but probably results from abnormal chemical reactions in the body which take place because of these infections. Reye's syndrome is not contagious. It most frequently affects children between 5 and 16 years of age.

The illness usually begins with vomiting, which lasts one to two days, and is followed by confusion and irrational behavior. At this point the child becomes irritable, aggressive, combative, and hostile.

Children with Reye's syndrome develop problems in the liver and brain. The illness can be diagnosed by a blood test that checks the liver. Hospitalization is necessary to allow close observation and treatment as needed. While Reye's syndrome is an extremely serious illness, most children recover completely without any long-lasting problems.

A Word about Aspirin and Reye's Syndrome

Recent research has linked Reye's syndrome with aspirin given to children who have had the flu or chicken pox. The cause of this relationship is presently unknown. Reye's syndrome is not caused by aspirin itself. Children who do not have influenza or chicken pox can take aspirin safely, in proper dosage. Once a child completely recovers from the flu or chicken pox, it is safe to give aspirin when necessary.

Many childhood illnesses resemble the flu. For example, it is practically impossible to distinguish a bad cold from a mild flu. For this reason it is not advisable to use aspirin to treat fever in any child under 16 years of age. If your child is very uncomfortable from a fever, you may want to treat the fever. In that situation you can safely use nonaspirin fever medicine (acetaminophen). The treatment of fever is discussed in detail in Chapter 26, "Fever."

37. *Sore Throats and Tonsillitis*

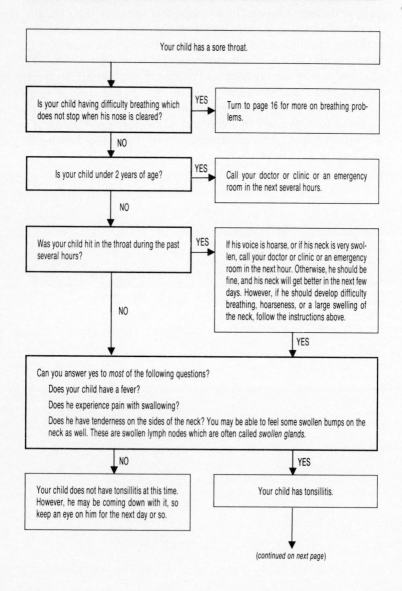

Your child has a sore throat.

Is your child having difficulty breathing which does not stop when his nose is cleared? — **YES** → Turn to page 16 for more on breathing problems.

NO

Is your child under 2 years of age? — **YES** → Call your doctor or clinic or an emergency room in the next several hours.

NO

Was your child hit in the throat during the past several hours? — **YES** → If his voice is hoarse, or if his neck is very swollen, call your doctor or clinic or an emergency room in the next hour. Otherwise, he should be fine, and his neck will get better in the next few days. However, if he should develop difficulty breathing, hoarseness, or a large swelling of the neck, follow the instructions above.

NO

YES

Can you answer yes to *most* of the following questions?

Does your child have a fever?

Does he experience pain with swallowing?

Does he have tenderness on the sides of the neck? You may be able to feel some swollen bumps on the neck as well. These are swollen lymph nodes which are often called *swollen glands*.

NO — Your child does not have tonsillitis at this time. However, he may be coming down with it, so keep an eye on him for the next day or so.

YES — Your child has tonsillitis.

(continued on next page)

(continued from preceding page)

Sore throats and tonsillitis are treated in much the same way as colds are. However, it is particularly important that your child keep drinking fluids so that he does not become dehydrated. Give plenty of cool, clear fluids which are *not* dietetic or sugar-free. Your child needs the sugar for energy to fight the infection and get better. Clear fluids include apple juice (half-strength for younger children) and other clear fruit juices and fruit drinks, flat ginger ale, water, ice desserts, and gelatin.

Call your doctor or clinic within the next day during regular office or phone hours and let the doctor know that your child has a sore throat. The doctor may want to get a throat culture to check for a strep throat (explained in detail in the chapter).

You may give your child nonaspirin fever medicine (acetaminophen) if he has a fever and seems uncomfortable. (Page 140 details fever treatment.)

Do not give your child any antibiotic without first checking with a doctor. This especially includes leftover prescriptions you have kept around the house. All leftover prescriptions should be thrown away.

The sore throat and other symptoms may last 1 to 2 weeks.

Call your doctor or clinic or an emergency room immediately if any of the following happens:

Your child becomes confused, disoriented, or delirious.

He becomes difficult to awaken.

He develops difficulty breathing which does not stop when his nose is cleared.

He develops signs of dehydration: he does not urinate at least once every 8 to 10 hours, his eyes become sunken, and his mouth becomes very dry.

He is acting very sick.

Call your doctor or clinic during regular office or phone hours if:

Your child's sore throat lasts more than 2 weeks.

He loses his voice.

You have any questions or concerns.

More about Sore Throats and Tonsillitis

Sore throats and tonsillitis are really the same thing. They are caused by an infection of the back of the throat.

Tonsillitis can occur at almost any age, but it is most common in young school-age children. There are two reasons for this. First, the body at this age has not yet fully built up its defenses against infection. Second, children are exposed to huge numbers of new germs as they meet many different children in school. Young school-age children are very susceptible to colds for the same reasons.

Sore throats are caused by viral infections in most cases. The viruses that cause sore throats are similar to the viruses that cause the common cold. There are no medicines at present that kill viruses. Antibiotics kill different types of germs, called *bacteria;* they have no effect on viruses. The best way to care for viral infections is to get plenty of rest, drink a sufficient amount of fluids, and treat fever if it is causing discomfort.

It is natural for children to have frequent sore throats. And it is not unusual for some children to have a sore throat several times a year, particularly in fall and winter. This is how the body builds its defenses against various types of viruses.

A sore throat usually is accompanied by a mild cough, runny nose, mild fever, and swollen "glands" in the neck. The back of the throat appears red, and the tonsils are enlarged. Usually at some point the tonsils will be covered spottily or entirely by a layer of white or yellow-white pus. This pus on the tonsils is not dangerous; it is an expected part of tonsillitis.

Swollen "glands" are actually swollen lymph nodes. Lymph nodes are present all the time, and are part of the body's defenses against infections. They usually go unnoticed until they become large and tender at times when they are fighting infection. Parents sometimes are concerned about cancer when they discover that their child has painfully swollen glands in the neck accompanying a sore throat. There is no cause for alarm; the swollen glands in this situation are *not* caused by leukemia or any other type of cancer.

Most sore throats caused by viral infection last 7 to 10 days. Children usually can handle sore throats without much difficulty as long as they drink sufficient fluids.

In rare cases tonsillitis becomes complicated by pus building up behind one tonsil. The collection of pus is called an *abscess*. It can cause a change in the voice, drooling, and breathing problems. Unlike pus *on* the tonsils, which is a normal reaction to tonsillitis, pus *behind* a tonsil is a serious problem that requires immediate medical attention. The abscess must be treated by antibiotics given through a vein in the arm for up to a week or more. Sometimes surgery is needed to drain the pus.

The medical term for sore throat or tonsillitis is *pharyngitis* (pronounced: fair un *jite* us); *pharynx* means "throat" and *itis* means "infection."

STREP THROAT

About 10 percent of the time, sore throats are caused by bacterial infection. The type of bacteria usually found is called *Streptococcus* (pronounced: strep tuh *cock* us). Strep throat is uncommon in children under 2 years of age. It is *impossible* for a doctor or anyone else to tell for sure from the symptoms and appearance of a sore throat whether it is strep throat. Only a throat culture can tell the difference between a sore throat caused by a virus and a sore throat caused by *Streptococcus* bacteria.

A throat culture is taken by swabbing the back of the throat with cotton. Unfortunately the person has to gag slightly to produce a good specimen. The cotton swab is then touched to a culture medium which allows the bacteria to grow. The culture medium, contained in a small covered dish, is placed in an incubator. If Streptococcus bacteria are present, the culture will detect them within 24 hours. Recently a new test has been developed which gives identification within minutes of streptococcal infection using throat swabs. This test is becoming widely available.

Strep throat is treated with antibiotics given by mouth for 10 days. They can be started up to a week after the infection hits and still be effective if the entire prescription is taken.

Removal of Tonsils and Adenoids

The tonsils and adenoids are located at the back of the throat. They are part of the body's defenses for fighting off colds, sore throats, and other infections. They may appear large in healthy children not because they are infected but because they grow at a faster rate than the rest of the body until age 13 or 14.

Tonsillectomy is the medical term for the surgical removal of both tonsils. The term *adenoidectomy* refers to removal of the adenoids. The surgical removal of the tonsils and adenoids at the same time is referred to as "T & A," (tonsillectomy and adenoidectomy).

Removing the tonsils and adenoids does not reduce the number or severity of colds and sore throats a child gets. It also does not reduce the number or severity of strep throats or ear infections. Removal does not improve hay fever or other allergies. There probably is no such thing as "chronic tonsillitis," and this should not be used as a reason to have a child undergo a tonsillectomy or adenoidectomy.

There are certain circumstances where removal of the tonsils and/or the adenoids is indicated, however. The adenoids may have to be removed if they block the breathing passages, or if they cause markedly nasal speech. The tonsils may have to be removed if they block the breathing passages, or if there are repeated episodes of pus behind the tonsils. Both the tonsils and adenoids may have to be removed in a certain type of heart disease, with certain breathing disorders, or with repeated pneumonia caused by swallowing problems.

Parents may feel a great need to do something besides giving careful support and attention to a child who suffers from repeated colds and sore throats. While this is under-standable, it is important to remember that repeated sore throats and colds are *natural events* during childhood. These repeated infections allow the growing child to build up his defenses, or *immunity*, to many different germs. If you have any further questions regarding tonsillectomy or adenoidec-tomy, discuss them with your doctor.

38. *Stomach Aches*

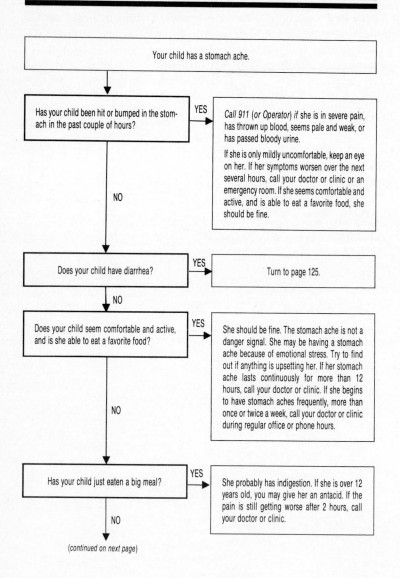

Your child has a stomach ache.

Has your child been hit or bumped in the stomach in the past couple of hours?

YES

Call 911 (or Operator) if she is in severe pain, has thrown up blood, seems pale and weak, or has passed bloody urine.

If she is only mildly uncomfortable, keep an eye on her. If her symptoms worsen over the next several hours, call your doctor or clinic or an emergency room. If she seems comfortable and active, and is able to eat a favorite food, she should be fine.

NO

Does your child have diarrhea?

YES

Turn to page 125.

NO

Does your child seem comfortable and active, and is she able to eat a favorite food?

YES

She should be fine. The stomach ache is not a danger signal. She may be having a stomach ache because of emotional stress. Try to find out if anything is upsetting her. If her stomach ache lasts continuously for more than 12 hours, call your doctor or clinic. If she begins to have stomach aches frequently, more than once or twice a week, call your doctor or clinic during regular office or phone hours.

NO

Has your child just eaten a big meal?

YES

She probably has indigestion. If she is over 12 years old, you may give her an antacid. If the pain is still getting worse after 2 hours, call your doctor or clinic.

NO

(continued on next page)

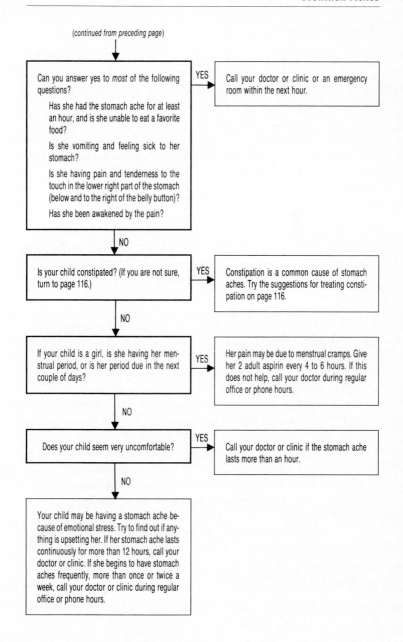

(continued from preceding page)

Can you answer yes to *most* of the following questions?

Has she had the stomach ache for at least an hour, and is she unable to eat a favorite food?

Is she vomiting and feeling sick to her stomach?

Is she having pain and tenderness to the touch in the lower right part of the stomach (below and to the right of the belly button)?

Has she been awakened by the pain?

YES → Call your doctor or clinic or an emergency room within the next hour.

NO

Is your child constipated? (If you are not sure, turn to page 116.)

YES → Constipation is a common cause of stomach aches. Try the suggestions for treating constipation on page 116.

NO

If your child is a girl, is she having her menstrual period, or is her period due in the next couple of days?

YES → Her pain may be due to menstrual cramps. Give her 2 adult aspirin every 4 to 6 hours. If this does not help, call your doctor during regular office or phone hours.

NO

Does your child seem very uncomfortable?

YES → Call your doctor or clinic if the stomach ache lasts more than an hour.

NO

Your child may be having a stomach ache because of emotional stress. Try to find out if anything is upsetting her. If her stomach ache lasts continuously for more than 12 hours, call your doctor or clinic. If she begins to have stomach aches frequently, more than once or twice a week, call your doctor or clinic during regular office or phone hours.

More about Stomach Aches

Stomach aches are a very common childhood problem. These pains usually last a short time and cause no difficulty. However, there are certain times when a stomach ache is an important signal that a child is developing a potentially serious problem. The map at the beginning of the chapter and the discussion below should help you decide when a stomach ache requires medical attention. The medical term for stomach ache is *abdominal pain*.

STOMACH ACHES CAUSED BY EMOTIONAL STRESS

In general, stress gives adults headaches and children stomach aches. Stomach aches caused by emotional stress are most common in the 5- to 10-year-old age group. They are felt in the area at or closely surrounding the belly button, and usually last one to two hours during any one attack.

Stomach pain caused by emotional stress is usually unrelated to a child's activities and bowel habits, but it can occur just before going to school or during meals. At times it may be possible to figure out the stressful situation triggering the stomach ache. Try to be sensitive to the stresses that may be affecting your child.

Frequently occurring stomach aches which interfere with activities at home and in school need to be investigated by a doctor. Nine times out of ten no medical problem will be found except emotional stress. In this situation, counseling is sometimes needed. Stress-related stomach aches often occur in families where there are other members who have tension headaches and stress-related intestinal complaints.

Children under 5 years old rarely have stomach aches caused by emotional stress. A stomach ache in this age group should be taken more seriously.

APPENDICITIS

Almost any time a child develops a stomach ache which seems to be more than trivial, parents will worry, "Is it appendicitis?" The map and this discussion address the issue directly. By following the map, you can tell when to consult a doctor for possible appendicitis.

Appendicitis most often occurs in people between the ages of 15 and 30 years, but essentially it can occur at any age. The typical appendicitis attack begins with a crampy stomach ache located throughout the abdominal area. This soon changes to pain and tenderness in the lower right area of the abdomen. Appendicitis is accompanied by a loss of appetite, nausea, and vomiting.

The diagnosis of appendicitis in a child can be very difficult to make for even the best-trained and most experienced doctors, because the typical symptoms of appendicitis in a teenager or young adult are often absent in children who have appendicitis. Still, you should be aware of the most important symptoms: a progressively worsening stomach ache followed by loss of appetite, nausea, and vomiting.

39. *Sunburn*

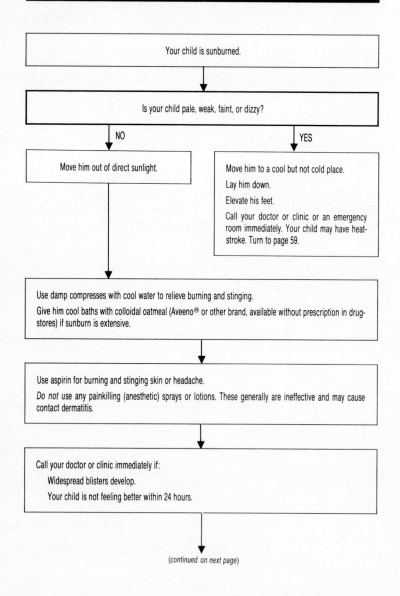

Your child is sunburned.

↓

Is your child pale, weak, faint, or dizzy?

NO ← → YES

NO: Move him out of direct sunlight.

YES: Move him to a cool but not cold place.

Lay him down.

Elevate his feet.

Call your doctor or clinic or an emergency room immediately. Your child may have heatstroke. Turn to page 59.

↓

Use damp compresses with cool water to relieve burning and stinging.

Give him cool baths with colloidal oatmeal (Aveeno® or other brand, available without prescription in drugstores) if sunburn is extensive.

↓

Use aspirin for burning and stinging skin or headache.

Do not use any painkilling (anesthetic) sprays or lotions. These generally are ineffective and may cause contact dermatitis.

↓

Call your doctor or clinic immediately if:

Widespread blisters develop.

Your child is not feeling better within 24 hours.

↓

(continued on next page)

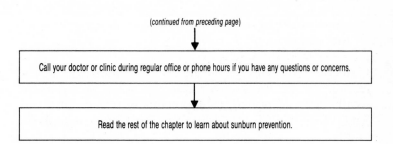

(continued from preceding page)

Call your doctor or clinic during regular office or phone hours if you have any questions or concerns.

Read the rest of the chapter to learn about sunburn prevention.

More about Sunburn

Sunburn is caused by exposure to ultraviolet (UV) light of a specific wavelength.

Children sunburn more easily than adults do. Fair-skinned, especially redheaded, persons also sunburn easily. Long-term overexposure to the sun can lead to many problems, including skin cancer, a prematurely aged appearance, loss of elasticity of the skin, and wrinkles.

Sunburn usually produces an initial painless redness of the skin which goes away after 1 to 2 hours. This is followed 6 to 12 hours later by the return of the redness plus a burning and stinging sensation. If the sunburn is severe enough, it will cause chills, headache, and an overall feeling of weakness and discomfort. In very severe cases heatstroke may occur.

PREVENTION OF SUNBURN

- *Use a sunscreen.* Sunscreens are now clearly labeled from 1 to 15, indicating the amount of protection they give; the higher the number, the more protection you get. For example, *15* means the sunscreen gives 15 times the natural protection your skin provides.

- *For children under 2 years of age,* use a 15-strength sunscreen.

- *For children over 2 years of age,* use at least an 8-strength sunscreen.

- *For children with very sun-sensitive skin,* use a sun-blocking agent such as zinc oxide or titanium oxide cream.

Apply sunscreen evenly and liberally to exposed areas. To ensure maximum protection, reapply sunscreen after swimming or vigorous exercise.

Infants and small children are very susceptible to sunburn. Infants should always wear sun hats when out in sunny weather. Avoid placing young infants in strong direct sunlight. When at the beach, keep your infant under an umbrella or otherwise in the shade.

Using T-shirts while in the water is a good way for older children to protect themselves from sunburn. Water acts as a reflector and can increase the risk of sunburn.

40. *Toddlers Who Say "No"*

You are having a terrible time trying to discipline your toddler.

Your child seems constantly to be testing you.

You are frustrated and feel pushed to the limit of your patience.

↓

Don't take it personally. (Really!)

Your child *is not* rejecting you.

Your child *is not* trying to get you angry.

Your child *is not* trying to aggravate you.

Your child *is* testing limits. This is how she learns about the world around her. You are both her guide to that world and her protector in that world. This is explained in further detail at the end of this chapter.

↓

If you feel overwhelmed, have your spouse, a friend, or a relative take care of your child for a while. Get out of the house by yourself for several hours.

↓

Do you feel frustrated to the point that you are afraid you cannot control yourself and you may strike or otherwise injure your child?

NO	YES
Read the rest of the chapter to learn specific ways to handle toddler behavior.	Put your child in her bedroom or somewhere where you know she will be safe. Then go and sit down, and call someone such as a close friend or relative. If all else fails, *call 911 (or Operator)* and ask for *Crisis Services*.

How to Handle a Toddler

Try these suggestions when you are with your toddler. They should help make your days more peaceful.

REMEMBER THE POWER OF "LET'S"

When you want your toddler to do something, do not ask her if she wants to do it; otherwise, be prepared to accept an answer of "no." If you ignore her response, you are only teaching her that her opinion does not count. Do not give your child options unless you want to.

Instead, tell your toddler in a nice way what is going to happen by using "let's." For example, "Anna, *let's* go upstairs and take a bath," or "Bill, *let's* go up to your room. It's bedtime."

GIVE CHOICES WHENEVER POSSIBLE

Teach your child to make choices, and help her develop a proper sense of self-worth and self-control by giving real choices as much as possible. Examples include asking your child if she wants milk or juice; letting your child pick out a shirt in the morning; letting her choose the book to be read, the game to be played, or the color crayon to be used. You will encounter countless similar situations throughout the day if you only look for the opportunities.

ALWAYS GIVE YOUR CHILD WARNING AHEAD OF TIME

Don't, if you can help it, suddenly spring something on toddlers. They are generally much more accepting of your decisions if they have time to digest them. For example, your toddler is playing and it is time for her bath. Tell her several minutes ahead of time that she will soon have to stop playing and get ready for her bath. Warn her again a minute or so before it's time to stop playing. When you finally want to take her in for the bath, she should be used to the idea and less likely to be upset.

ACKNOWLEDGE BUT DO NOT INDULGE TEMPER TANTRUMS

If your child becomes upset at a decision you have made, let her know you are aware of her anger but explain your position. Example: I have just told my daughter Leah that it's time for bed. She starts to cry and throws herself on the ground. I pick her up, carry her upstairs in my arms, and tell her, "Leah, I know you do not want to go to bed, but it is bedtime. Tomorrow is another day, I'll see you first thing in the morning, and we're going to have lots of fun."

DON'T ARGUE WITH TODDLERS

There is nothing to be gained in arguing with toddlers. Explain to them what is going to happen and then implement your plan. As always, acknowledge that you understand that they are upset and explain why things have to be that way.

DISCIPLINE SWIFTLY AND BRIEFLY

When a toddler engages in behavior that is either dangerous or totally unacceptable, discipline is indicated. Such behaviors include hitting, biting, throwing objects, standing on tables, running into the street, spitting food at others, and drawing on walls.

In all of the above situations a brief spank on the bottom is appropriate. *Explain* to your child why she was punished. Immediately following an incident, you should ask your toddler to explain to you or your spouse why she was punished.

Use "Time-Out" as a Form of Discipline

"Time-out" is a very effective way to discipline a toddler. It works like this: you have a place in the house where your child must sit for a brief period of time if she has done something unacceptable. For example, your toddler has just thrown a truck at her infant brother, narrowly missing her target. You swiftly pick her up, and let her know that what she did was dangerous and wrong. You then put her on a chair in the corner of the room, and tell her she must sit there for five minutes. Don't stay with her. Resume your regular activities as much as possible, checking only occasionally to make sure she is still sitting.

Remove Bones of Contention

If you do not want your child to play with your necktie and get it all full of spaghetti sauce, take it off and put it out of reach. I am sure you can think of many similar examples. Child-proofing serves two purposes: not only does it remove items which are dangerous to your child, it also removes objects which you may wish to protect and not argue about all the time.

Use Distraction and Substitution

Distraction and substitution may work in many situations. If your child wants to grab and rip up your Sunday paper, give her Saturday's to demolish. Or consider that she may be asking you to pay attention to her. If that is the case, read the comics to her.

Emphasize What Your Toddler Can Do, Not What She Cannot Do

Re-stating limits in a positive way can be a very helpful technique when your toddler wants to do something she shouldn't. This often comes up when a toddler wants to do what her brother or sister is doing.

For example, our 23-month-old, Anna, was trying to get into a bouncing chair that we had brought down for our 5-month-old, Leah, to use. Anna had used this when she was an infant. She now was trying to climb into the chair. I explained to her briefly that she was now a big girl and this chair was for Leah. She did not accept my explanation and began to cry when I told her again, firmly, not to get into the chair.

At this point my wife entered the scene. She picked up Anna and skillfully started talking about all the people in the family—cousins, aunts, and uncles—who were too big to use the chair. Anna, too, started naming the "big people," and after a short time the issue had passed.

SET RIGID BOUNDARIES AROUND A FLEXIBLE ENVIRONMENT

This may sound like a contradiction, but it really isn't. Children at all ages require age-appropriate freedoms in order to explore and learn about their world. Parents must set a stage for their children that is safe but not overly confining.

Toddlers are constantly forging into the world. They are like a windup toy that keeps bouncing off an obstacle until it makes its way around it.

Boundaries of acceptable behavior must be clear to your child. The boundaries must be defined constantly and consistently. This will be reassuring to your child; it will give her confidence to explore the world because she will be taking off from a stable environment which you have constructed. This is what I mean by being *rigid*.

We parents must be attuned to what is appropriate for each age of development. For example, what can you appropriately expect of a 2-year-old, and what is an excessive demand for a child of this age? What demands are unfair, or employed simply because they are convenient or suitable to our adult needs?

It is unreasonable to expect a 2-year-old to sit through a

two-hour movie, so don't take her to one. It is reasonable, on the other hand, to take your 12-year-old.

It is unfair to expect a 3-year-old to sit next to a birthday cake without plunging her hands into the icing. Your 10-year-old should be old enough to wait.

Do not expect your 20-month-old to understand why she cannot eat peanuts. Simply refrain from serving them in her presence. These minor sacrifices will soon—and, you may often find, sadly—no longer be necessary.

In short, there are daily situations where you must be willing to be *flexible* and allow your child to act her age.

41. *Vomiting*

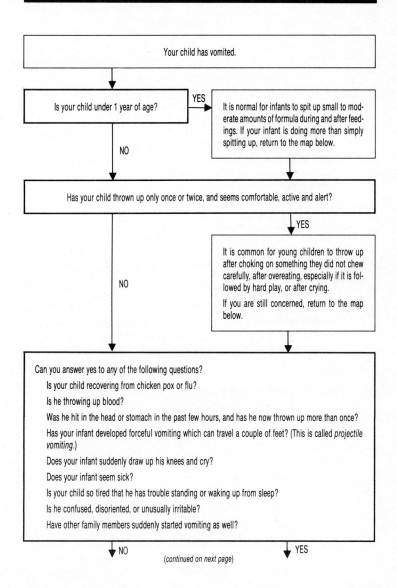

Your child has vomited.

Is your child under 1 year of age?

YES → It is normal for infants to spit up small to moderate amounts of formula during and after feedings. If your infant is doing more than simply spitting up, return to the map below.

NO

Has your child thrown up only once or twice, and seems comfortable, active and alert?

YES → It is common for young children to throw up after choking on something they did not chew carefully, after overeating, especially if it is followed by hard play, or after crying.

If you are still concerned, return to the map below.

NO

Can you answer yes to *any* of the following questions?

Is your child recovering from chicken pox or flu?

Is he throwing up blood?

Was he hit in the head or stomach in the past few hours, and has he now thrown up more than once?

Has your infant developed forceful vomiting which can travel a couple of feet? (This is called *projectile vomiting*.)

Does your infant suddenly draw up his knees and cry?

Does your infant seem sick?

Is your child so tired that he has trouble standing or waking up from sleep?

Is he confused, disoriented, or unusually irritable?

Have other family members suddenly started vomiting as well?

NO **YES**

(continued on next page)

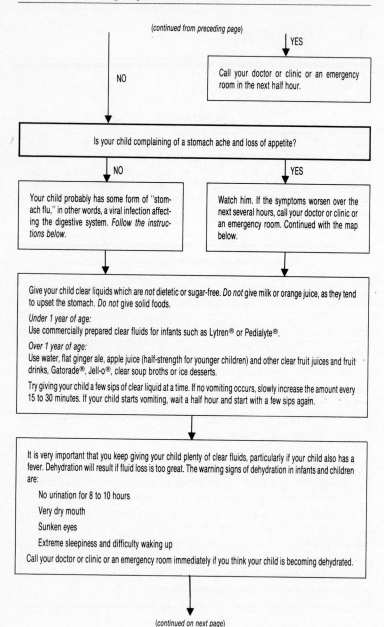

(continued from preceding page)

YES

NO

Call your doctor or clinic or an emergency room in the next half hour.

Is your child complaining of a stomach ache and loss of appetite?

NO

YES

Your child probably has some form of "stomach flu," in other words, a viral infection affecting the digestive system. *Follow the instructions below.*

Watch him. If the symptoms worsen over the next several hours, call your doctor or clinic or an emergency room. Continued with the map below.

Give your child clear liquids which are *not* dietetic or sugar-free. *Do not* give milk or orange juice, as they tend to upset the stomach. *Do not* give solid foods.

Under 1 year of age:
Use commercially prepared clear fluids for infants such as Lytren® or Pedialyte®.

Over 1 year of age:
Use water, flat ginger ale, apple juice (half-strength for younger children) and other clear fruit juices and fruit drinks, Gatorade®, Jell-o®, clear soup broths or ice desserts.

Try giving your child a few sips of clear liquid at a time. If no vomiting occurs, slowly increase the amount every 15 to 30 minutes. If your child starts vomiting, wait a half hour and start with a few sips again.

It is very important that you keep giving your child plenty of clear fluids, particularly if your child also has a fever. Dehydration will result if fluid loss is too great. The warning signs of dehydration in infants and children are:

No urination for 8 to 10 hours

Very dry mouth

Sunken eyes

Extreme sleepiness and difficulty waking up

Call your doctor or clinic or an emergency room immediately if you think your child is becoming dehydrated.

(continued on next page)

(continued from preceding page)

↓

You may give your child nonaspirin fever medicine (acetaminophen) if he has a fever and seems uncomfortable. (See page 144 for proper dosage.) Otherwise, *do not give your child any medicines*, including aspirin, unless directed to do so by your doctor.

↓

If your child starts getting better after 24 hours, do the following:

Under 1 year of age:
Start with half-strength formula and work him back to full-strength over the next few days. If he also has had diarrhea, start with half-strength soy-based formula (Prosobee® or Isomil®) or quarter-strength regular formula. Slowly increase the strength of the formula over the next 2 to 3 days. You should not have to continue the soy-based formula for more than 5 to 7 days.

Over 1 year of age:
Begin with the following foods:

Bananas	Bland crackers such as Saltines	Dry toast
Rice	Carrots (raw or cooked)	
Rice cereal without milk	Peeled apples or applesauce	

Keep giving the clear liquids, but taper the amount as he gets better. Keep him off milk for 5 to 7 days. Slowly bring him back to a regular diet.

↓

Call your doctor or clinic during regular office or phone hours if:

Your child is not getting better after 24 to 36 hours.

You have any questions or concerns.

More about Vomiting

Vomiting in children is a common problem that has many different causes. The most common cause is a viral infection which may cause your child to have fever, an upset stomach, and diarrhea as well as vomiting. This is a temporary illness which requires adjustments in diet as outlined on the map.

The preceding map will also help you decide when to be concerned about your child's vomiting and when to seek medical advice or care.

42. *Warts*

Warts are small bumps or lumps found on the skin. They are not dangerous. Warts most commonly occur on the face, top of the fingers, back of the hands, palms, soles, elbows, and knees. They are usually skin-colored but can be tan or white. A person can have one wart or several. A wart can have either a flat or irregular surface.

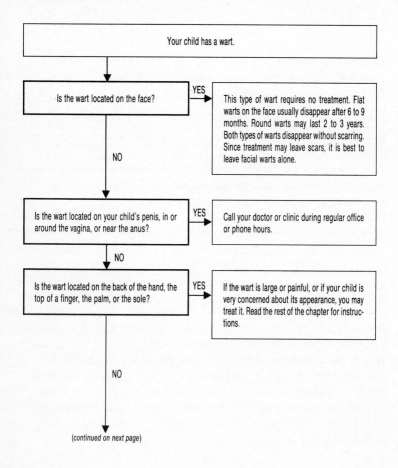

Your child has a wart.

Is the wart located on the face?

YES → This type of wart requires no treatment. Flat warts on the face usually disappear after 6 to 9 months. Round warts may last 2 to 3 years. Both types of warts disappear without scarring. Since treatment may leave scars, it is best to leave facial warts alone.

NO

Is the wart located on your child's penis, in or around the vagina, or near the anus?

YES → Call your doctor or clinic during regular office or phone hours.

NO

Is the wart located on the back of the hand, the top of a finger, the palm, or the sole?

YES → If the wart is large or painful, or if your child is very concerned about its appearance, you may treat it. Read the rest of the chapter for instructions.

NO

(continued on next page)

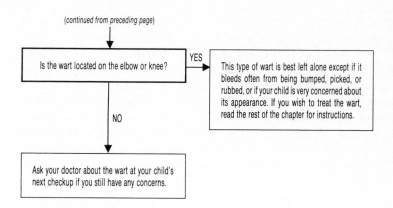

(continued from preceding page)

Is the wart located on the elbow or knee? — **YES** → This type of wart is best left alone except if it bleeds often from being bumped, picked, or rubbed, or if your child is very concerned about its appearance. If you wish to treat the wart, read the rest of the chapter for instructions.

NO

Ask your doctor about the wart at your child's next checkup if you still have any concerns.

More about Warts

A wart is caused by a mild viral infection of the skin which causes the skin to fold upon itself in an irregular way. Even though warts are caused by viruses, most types of warts are not very contagious. It is not necessary to isolate a child who has warts.

Warts can be located anywhere on the skin, but they are most commonly found on the palms and soles. Warts located here are termed *palmar warts* and *plantar warts,* respectively. Warts can also appear on the face, the back of the hands, and the back of the fingers.

Very irregular and branching warts, which look like small cauliflowers, can occur on the penis, in and around the vagina, and around the anus. They deserve special attention because they are passed on by sexual contact, and are therefore a form of venereal disease. In children less than 12 or 13 years old, genital or anal warts should be assumed to have been caused by sexual abuse unless proved otherwise. This is an upsetting but very important topic. For more information about sexual abuse, turn to Chapter 18, "Child Abuse."

Warts often go away by themselves without leaving a scar. Often it is best to leave them alone, particularly warts on the face. Large and painful warts should be treated; plantar warts can be particularly painful. You might also consider treatment if your child is very self-conscious about a wart.

Warts can be treated in many different ways. Using a 40 percent salicylic acid plaster as described below is safe, inexpensive, and painless. Duofilm® is used almost identically, but you need a prescription to get it. Sometimes it is most convenient to have your doctor freeze a wart with liquid nitrogen. Methods such as surgery and electrosurgery should be avoided, since the resulting scar may become more of a problem than the wart. A wart sometimes regrows into the scar.

No method of treatment is perfect. Warts will return about 25 percent of the time no matter what form of treatment is used.

How to Treat Warts

The preceding map tells you when to treat warts and when to leave them alone. The instructions below tell you how to treat warts.

Warts can be treated at home with 40 percent salicylic acid plaster, which is not a prescription medication. It's a mild acid which slowly dissolves warts. Avoid using this medicine with preschoolers and infants, because they may pick at the plaster and put it in their mouths.

Listed below are specific instructions for using 40 percent salicylic acid plaster on warts. The medicine comes in thin square sheets which can be cut with a scissors. A small piece of the plaster is applied to the wart daily as follows:

1. Apply enough plaster to cover the entire wart. The sticky brown side goes against the wart. Use a scissors to cut the plaster so it fits. Try not to get any plaster on the surrounding normal skin. You may protect the surrounding skin with petroleum jelly.

2. Cover the plaster securely with adhesive tape. Wrap the tape around the edge of the hand or foot if the wart is on the palm or sole.

3. Keep the plaster on all day and night and remove it only before applying new medication. It can be left on for up to 24 hours or until the next bath or shower. Avoid getting the plaster wet.

4. Change the plaster as follows:
   - Remove the old adhesive tape and plaster.
   - Rub away the surface of the wart for a couple of minutes with an emery board, nail file, or pumice stone. This should not be painful.
   - Wet the area for at least five minutes. This may be done in the bath. Dry the area with a towel. Reapply the plaster following step 1.

5. If the area becomes painful, stop the treatment for two or three days. If the pain stops, try again. Call your doctor or clinic during regular office or phone hours if the area is still painful or if pain returns when the medication is restarted.

6. A small amount of bleeding from the wart may occur. You can continue using the plaster in this situation. If bleeding occurs frequently, call your doctor or clinic during regular office or phone hours.

7. Be patient. Treatment may take several weeks. Over time the wart will slowly wear away. Stop treatment when the wart has completely disappeared.

III. *Prevention*

43. *Prevention of Accidents*

The Importance of Prevention

Accidents account for more deaths among American children than the combined fatalities from these five leading causes of death: cancer, heart disease, birth defects, pneumonia, and meningitis! Motor-vehicle accidents are the greatest single cause of death in children and young adults in this country.

The impact of accidental injury and death is staggering. Every day across the country almost 3,000 children seek medical attention for an accidental injury. Of these 3,000 children, almost 300 will be seriously maimed or crippled for life, and almost 30 will die. That translates into 100,000 children suffering serious lifelong disability, and 10,000 accidental childhood deaths annually. *All of which is preventable!*

It is for this reason that accident prevention is stressed throughout this book. The challenge for the 1980s and beyond, for parents, educators, physicians, and all those concerned with the health and welfare of children in this country, is to reduce the toll that accidental injury and death takes on our children. What can be done about this problem? This chapter will give specific instructions that will enable you to construct the safest possible environment for your child.

While accident statistics are alarming, it is important to keep in mind that this is not a reason to be overprotective. Childhood is a time of learning which requires the child to explore the world in which she lives. Children should not develop an exaggerated fear of injury. Following prudent measures lets you create a supervised environment for younger children. As your child grows, she should be learning the principles of safety. Having learned these principles, she will be able to supervise herself. This will enable her to explore her world fully and enjoy her childhood years with a minimum of risk to her health and safety.

The American Academy of Pediatrics has recommended five steps as some of the most effective measures parents can take to avoid injuries in their children:

1. Using approved car restraints for children.

2. Installing smoke detectors in the home which protect all children's sleeping quarters.

3. Turning down the hot-water tank to a safe temperature— 120° to 130° Fahrenheit (49° to 54° Celsius). This is the "warm" setting or just above the "warm" setting, at most.

4. Installing window and stairway guards and gates to prevent falls.

5. Keeping a 1-ounce bottle of syrup of ipecac in the house, and being ready to use it upon the advice of the local poison control center. Ipecac is available without prescription, and can be found in most drugstores.

These instructions will be covered further in the next several pages. Specific topics include: car safety; home safety, which deals with the prevention of burns, electrical injuries, falls, choking, and poisoning; bicycle safety; water safety; toy safety; and animal safety. In addition, throughout this book, at the end of each chapter, there is usually a discussion of safety and prevention.

The Risks as Your Child Grows

When you are trying to prevent accidents, it helps to know when and where accidents are likely to occur. It also helps to know the different risks to expect as your child grows older. This information will help you effectively apply prevention techniques.

Childhood injuries most often occur in family cars, at home, on bicycles, in water, and around animals. Boys are involved in accidents much more often than girls are. Injuries peak during the summer months and hit a low point during the winter.

As children grow, they encounter specific hazards and risks at each age. The risks encountered depend upon the abilities and activities of children at each stage of development. For children of all ages, however, automobiles remain the greatest cause of injury and death.

FROM BIRTH TO 6 MONTHS OF AGE

Young infants learn to lift their heads and soon after will be able to wiggle around and fall off things. They will also be able to reach for dangerous objects. Injuries at this age most commonly result from:

Automobile accidents	Burns
Falls	Choking

FROM 7 TO 12 MONTHS OF AGE

At this age infants begin to roll over, crawl, sit, and stand. Some infants will be able to walk with support and even climb. They will be able to grasp for almost anything, and whatever they grab will usually find its way quickly into their mouths. Injuries at this age most commonly result from:

Automobile accidents	Poisoning
Falls	Choking
Burns	

FROM 1 TO 2 YEARS OF AGE

At this age children will be entering the *most accident-prone* stage of their lives. They will be able to walk, run, climb, jump, and, above all else, *explore* everything. Toddlers move fast, and you have to "watch them like a hawk." Injuries at this age most commonly result from:

Automobile accidents	Burns	Falls
Poisoning	Drowning	
Choking	Animal bites	

FROM 2 TO 4 YEARS OF AGE

Children at this age are moving and learning fast. They will now be able to run, jump, ride tricycles, and use tools. Injuries at this age most commonly result from:

Automobile accidents   Drowning
Falls   Animal bites
Burns   Poisoning

FROM 4 YEARS OF AGE TO THE TEENAGE YEARS

As children grow, they will be exposed continually to household appliances, tools, and machines. During the school years they will be tempted increasingly by dares and challenges. Over competitiveness, recklessness, and poor preparation play a role in sports injuries.

A teenage boy is four times as likely as a teenage girl to suffer an accidental death. Injuries associated with drug and alcohol abuse are common at this age. Injuries at this age most commonly result from:

Automobile accidents   Drowning
Bicycle accidents   Sports accidents

Car Safety

Traveling by car should always be a safe and enjoyable experience for you and your family. Unfortunately, motor-vehicle accidents are the greatest cause of death and injury in children and young adults in this country. Young infants are particularly vulnerable, and lap-held infants are at the greatest risk of all. One out of every forty children born in the United States this year will die from an automobile injury before he or she is 25 years old.

Great care, common sense, and good judgment should always be used when you travel by car. The *safest* place in the car for your infant, toddler, or young child is in his car safety seat.

Can you answer yes to *any* of the following questions?

Is your child less than 5 years old?

Is he less than 44 inches tall?

Does he weigh less than 45 pounds?

(Remember, it is the size not the age that counts. A small 6-year-old should still be in a safety seat.)

NO

YES

He no longer needs a safety seat. However, he should always wear a seat belt. Please note that children who are less than 55 inches tall should *not* use a shoulder strap because, for them, the strap increases the risk of neck injury. You can buckle the belt portion around your child and pass the strap behind him.

He should always be in a safety seat when traveling in any car. In most states it is illegal not to use one.

There are four types of safety seats: one for infants who weigh less than 20 pounds (up to 9 to 12 months of age), a standard type for toddlers and young children, a booster-type seat for toddlers and young children, and an adjustable model which can fit infants, toddlers, and young children.

Before buying a safety seat, take it out to your car and make sure it fits and is easy to use.

Remember, probably the *single most important thing* you can ever do for your child's safety is to buy and properly use a car safety seat. If you still don't believe this, read the rest of the chapter.

SOME ANSWERS TO QUESTIONS COMMONLY ASKED ABOUT SAFETY SEATS

1. *How do I get my child to sit still in a safety seat?* Newborn infants should be taken home from the hospital in car seats. Thereafter, *every time* your child rides in the car he should be in a safety seat. Children who always use car seats will be accustomed to sitting safely buckled. For older infants and toddlers, pleasant activities such as listening to parents talking or singing will help them learn to enjoy traveling in the car. A few small toys or a favorite blanket can also help. *Seeing parents buckle up each time makes a big difference too.*

2. *Why can't I just hold my little baby in my lap?* A mother holding a 10-pound baby in a car moving 30 miles per hour would have to be able to lift 300 pounds if she wanted to stop her baby from flying out of her arms in the event of a collision. The baby would act like a missile and would either be smashed into the windshield or would be crushed between the dashboard and his mother. Holding a baby in your arms or on your lap is clearly unsafe.

3. *Why can't I just use the seat belts for my young children?* Seat belts are designed for adults. They do not work well for young children because children have a higher center of gravity, a relatively lower neck, and undeveloped hip bones. For these reasons young children can be seriously injured wearing seat belts designed for use by older children and adults.

4. *Isn't it dangerous for my child to be "trapped" inside a car seat?* No. Your child's chance of injury or death is *50 times greater* if he is thrown from the car through a window or open door.

5. *Do safety seats really work?* Yes, they do work. It is estimated that at least 9 out of 10 deaths from automobile accidents could have been prevented by using safety seats.

Also, two-thirds of all injuries could have been prevented by using them.

DIFFERENT MODELS OF SAFETY SEATS

Since 1981, all child safety seats sold in the United States have been required to meet minimum federal safety regulations. However, all seats are not equally easy to install, equally easy to use, or equally comfortable for your child.

There are four types of seats: one for infants only, a standard type for toddlers and young children, a booster-type seat for toddlers and young children, and an adjustable type.

The adjustable model may appear to be the most practical and economical for many parents. However, the infant-only seats do make it easy to carry an infant in and out of the car. They also can be used in the home as an infant seat. For these reasons some parents might find the extra expense of an infant-only seat to be a good investment.

The booster-type seat resembles a restaurant booster seat. It has an abdominal piece or bar through or over which the lap belt passes. They are easy to use, and are usually well tolerated by older kids (3- to 5-year-olds). Booster-type seats have minimum weight and height requirements which vary (i.e., the child should be at least 30 pounds and 33 inches).

Certain child safety seats have a tether that anchors the seat to the car and works in tandem with the seat belt. The tether must be bolted to the car frame. This often requires that you have a mechanic install a bolt in your car. A properly installed tethered seat will provide more head restraint in case of a severe crash. This could be especially important in a small car.

There are many ways to learn about the specific models of car seats available before you make a purchase. Other parents with older children who have used car seats since the time their children were infants are probably the best people to ask. You can also ask your doctor, local hospital, or local department of motor vehicles.

Child safety seats range in price anywhere from about $20 to $80 or more. As their children grow, many families rotate car seats among each other to help keep costs down. Also, certain organizations will loan seats for a nominal fee. A hospital's infant nursery, your local health department, the state highway office, or your doctor can help you find out if this service is available in your community.

In many states young children and infants by law must be in car safety seats at all times. In 1978 Tennessee became the first state in the Union to mandate the use of child-restraint devices. Since the introduction of this law in Tennessee, the number of childhood deaths from automobile injuries has dropped by more than half in that state. Many other states have enacted similar legislation over the past several years.

Last of all, remember that the time to start using a car safety seat is from the beginning. *Every* newborn baby should ride home from the hospital in a car seat. Make the first ride a safe one!

Home Safety

The home is second only to the automobile as the place where children are most frequently injured. Prevention should be focused on the following types of injuries: burns, electrical injuries, falls, choking, and poisoning. *Toddlers* are at the greatest risk for all of these injuries. *Toddler-proofing* a house is probably a more accurate term than *child-proofing*.

PREVENTION OF BURNS

- *Make sure your home has working smoke detectors* that protect all sleeping areas. Check your smoke detector's batteries frequently.

- Have at least two working fire extinguishers in your home

at all times. They should be within easy reach. The kitchen and your bedroom are good places for storing fire extinguishers.

- Keep your hot-water heater at a safe temperature—120° to 130° Fahrenheit (49° to 54° Celsius). Turn the setting to "warm" or just above "warm," at most. At this setting the heater will still provide you with water hot enough for comfortable baths and showers. Not only will this prevent scalds, it will also help you save on your utility bills.

- Keep drain cleaners and other dangerous chemicals out of reach. A locked cabinet is the best place for them. *Under the sink is the worst place for them.*

- Never eat, drink, hold, or carry anything hot when holding an infant or child. Never smoke when holding an infant or child.

- When preparing meals, make sure that your child is playing safely outside the kitchen and is not under foot. Hot drinks, liquids, foods, and grease can all cause serious burns. Also, make sure that pot handles are always turned *inward* so that they cannot be tipped over by a curious toddler.

- Make sure that cups and other containers containing hot liquids are safely out of reach, and are not near the edge of tables and counters.

- Have a practice fire drill with all family members at least once a year.

Prevention of Electrical Injuries

- If you have infants and young children, make sure all open electric outlets are covered with safety caps.

- As your infant begins to crawl and explore, make sure all electric cords are out of biting range.

- Educate older children to the dangers of high-power lines, high-voltage transformer stations, and the third rail of electrified train tracks.

- Always make sure that electric appliances are properly installed. This is particularly important for appliances requiring heavy-duty lines, such as stoves, washers, and driers.

- Do not overload household lines with multiple adapters, and never place a penny under a blown fuse.

PREVENTION OF FALLS

- *Never* walk away from an infant who is on a changing table or any other high place. Infants are never too young to wiggle and fall.

- Starting when your child is around 6 months of age, use restraints on stairways and doors.

- Keep infants and toddlers out of rooms where they might climb and hurt themselves.

- Cover or temporarily store all sharp-edged furniture.

- Use window guards on all windows above the first floor.

PREVENTION OF CHOKING

- Never leave small objects in an infant's or small child's reach even for a moment.

- Never feed your infant or young child *large or hard pieces of food*, especially hard candy and large pieces of meat.

- Never feed peanuts, bacon, or popcorn to children under the age of 6 or 7 years. Peanuts are very slippery and can pass easily into a child's windpipe. Bacon breaks into small slivers that can travel easily into the lungs. Popcorn is very light and can be sucked easily into a child's lungs.

- Gum should not be given to children under 6 or 7 years of

age. Young children can choke easily on gum because they can't chew well enough yet.

• Never give children uninflated balloons to play with. They can be very dangerous, as they can be sucked down the windpipe easily.

PREVENTION OF POISONING

Poisoning most often occurs in the kitchen, bathroom, basement workroom, and garage. Medicines and household materials such as paints, cleaners, solvents, and polish usually are involved.

Young children will put *anything and everything in their mouths*. You must make your home safe by putting medicines and dangerous household products high up, *out of reach, out of sight, in child-proof containers*. It is best to lock up all medicines, including nonprescription medications such as aspirin and nonaspirin pain and fever medicine (acetaminophen). Make sure that there are no dangerous cleaning materials under your sink, and that your garage and basement are also safe.

Find out the telephone number of the nearest poison control center, and write it next to your telephone and in the space provided in this book in Chapter 15, "Poisoning."

There is no such thing as a "universal antidote." Many of the instructions listed on containers of hazardous material are out of date and incorrect. Always check first with your doctor or local poison control center before giving your child anything following an ingestion of a poisonous substance.

Buy a bottle of ipecac (pronounced: *ip* ih kack) and store it in a safe place with your other medicines. Ipecac can be purchased without prescription and is available in most drugstores. This medicine is used in certain situations to make a person vomit and expel poisonous material from the stomach. Ipecac can be dangerous in certain situations, however. So *never* give your child ipecac or anything else before speaking to your doctor or local poison control center.

When you are visiting relatives (especially older family members) or when they are visiting you be sure to ask if they have any medicines around the house or with them. If so, be sure to store the medicines safely out of the reach of small children. Remember, pocketbooks often contain medicines. Many an accidental poisoning has resulted from a curious toddler eating the "candy" she has found in Grandma's purse.

First-Aid Kit

Some families like to have two kits: a smaller one for the car, and a larger one in their home. The safety kit should be stored in an area safely out of children's reach, but easily accessible to adults. You can use a tackle box or small tool box. The kit should be locked when not in use.

A household first-aid kit should include the items listed below:

- Plenty of adhesive bandages of various sizes.
- Several rolls of different size adhesive tape. Clear adhesive tape works well and is easy to use. It can be used to secure adhesive bandages which may otherwise fall off.
- Scissors, tweezers, and safety pins.
- Matches to sterilize the tweezers or pins used to remove splinters.
- Plenty of sterile gauze pads: 2" × 2", and 4" × 4".
- A bar of plain white soap.
- Iodine antiseptic solution for cleaning cuts.
- Aspirin and nonaspirin pain reliever (acetaminophen). Both children's and adult tablets should be included.
- Syrup of ipecac. (Always check with a poison control center or emergency room before using ipecac.)
- A thermometer.
- A pad and pencil.

Bicycle Safety

The bicycle is at the top of the Consumer Product Safety Commission's list of hazardous products. Each year over 1 million bicycle-related injuries occur in the United States. One in three of these injuries is serious enough to require a visit to an emergency room. Head injury is the most common injury suffered by young bicycle riders.

CHOOSING A BICYCLE FOR YOUR CHILD

A bicycle should be carefully chosen to suit your child's size and age.

Seat.   Should be no higher than your child's hips.

Pedals.   Your child's feet should reach the pedals without the aid of blocks. Avoid plastic pedals. Use rubber-treaded or metal pedals with serrated edges.

Handlebars.   Your child should be able to reach the handlebars easily when sitting on the bicycle seat.

Brakes.   Young children's bicycles should have foot brakes. Hand brakes require too much strength and coordination for kids under 11 or 12 years of age.

All bicycles should have retroreflectors on the front and rear. For night riding (older children only), a headlight in front and taillight or red reflector in back are necessary; in some states they are required by law. Reflecting tape on the bicycle is a good idea. Use white in the front and red in the back. The rider should always wear light-colored clothing. Reflecting clothing is also an excellent idea.

Boys should use bicycles that do not have the gearshifts on the crossbar; these can cause genital injury.

Keep the bicycle in good condition. Check the brakes regularly and be familiar with how they work. Regular, expert maintenance is a must for safe riding. An experienced, qualified person should do complicated work.

TIPS FOR SAFE BICYCLING

• Always wear a safety helmet. Children in carrier seats should wear safety helmets at all times.

• Learn and obey all traffic rules, traffic signs, and traffic signals.

• Use bicycle paths whenever possible.

• When riding on the sidewalk, give pedestrians the right of way.

• When riding in the street, ride with the flow of traffic on the right side. Never ride against the flow of traffic.

• Never ride on streets where there is heavy automobile traffic.

• Walk—do not ride—the bicycle across busy intersections and around corners when you are making a left turn.

• Avoid riding in wet weather.

• Never ride with two people on one bike (except with children in carrier seats). Balancing is difficult, and vision can be blocked. Passengers commonly suffer injuries of the feet and legs from the spokes.

• Never ride barefoot. Wear rubber-soled shoes and keep feet on the pedals.

• Carrier seats should have footrests, foot guards, foot straps, and seat belts. Carrier seats are advisable only for infants and young children. As mentioned above, helmets should be worn by children riding in carrier seats.

Water Safety

Several guidelines concerning water safety are given in Chapter 7, "Drowning."

Toy Safety

Toys are not only a source of entertainment and amusement, they are also educational. Toys can be dangerous, however, if they are poorly designed or poorly constructed or if they are used by children of the wrong age. For example, a game of marbles is fine for a 10-year-old, but marbles left on the floor are potentially lethal to a toddler who might put them in his mouth. When purchasing toys, pay close attention to the age recommendations of the manufacturer.

The table below will help you decide which toys are safe for your child.

Unsafe and Safe Toys

Child's Age	Unsafe Toys	Safe Toys
Under 2 years	Toys small enough to swallow Flammable toys Toys with small, removable parts Stuffed animals with glass or button eyes	Books Brightly colored beads on a strong cord Washable squeak toys Large, soft balls Stuffed animals *without* glass or button eyes Blocks with rounded corners Push-and-pull toys (Make sure the cord is not long enough to go around your child's neck.) Sturdy rattles
2 to 3 years	Marbles, beads, coins Flammable toys Toys with sharp edges Toys with small, removable parts	Books Wooden animals Large crayons Rocking toys Sturdy cars and wagons Large pegboards

(*continued*)

Unsafe and Safe Toys (*Continued*)

Child's Age	Unsafe Toys	Safe Toys
3 to 6 years	Sharp or cutting toys Flammable costumes Electric toys Shooting games Poisonous paint sets Ill-balanced tricycles or wagons	Books Nonelectric trains Building blocks Blackboards and dustless chalk Modeling clay Simple construction sets Paints and paint books Child-size sports equipment
6 to 12 years	Nonapproved electric toys (Make sure all electric toys have the Underwriters Laboratory, or UL, seal or approval.) Sharp-edged tools Poorly made sports equipment Shooting toys: air rifles in particular Conductible kites All-terrain cycles, or ATCs (ATCs are extremely dangerous; they can cause severe, even lethal, injury.) Trampolines (unsafe at any age)	Books Workbench and lightweight tools for younger children Construction sets Hobby materials UL-approved electric toys, used under supervision Well-constructed sports equipment Robot toys

Animal Safety

Children are more likely to be bitten by animals than are adults. Children are generally friendlier to animals, and their small size makes them less capable of defending themselves.

Animal-safety measures are listed below.

• Avoid all unfamiliar, wild, sick, or injured animals.

• Do not take in stray animals.

- Have your own pet or pets vaccinated.
- Report any unfamiliar, wild, sick, or injured animal to the police.
- Do not let children break up an animal fight even if it involves your own pet. An adult should use a rake, broom, or other object to separate the animals.

44. *Immunizations (Shots)*

The terms *baby shots, immunizations,* and *vaccines* all refer to the same thing: tiny doses of germs or germ products which are given to strengthen the body's defenses. The body's system of defenses against infection is called the *immune system.*

The first time a person's immune system is exposed to a germ during an infection, it builds a specific defense to fight off that specific germ. The next time the person is exposed to that same germ, the immune system usually will prevent another infection. Vaccines work because they stimulate the immune system without causing a serious infection.

Infants and children are helped by vaccines because their immune systems are young and have not yet been exposed to most germs. Older children and adults also may require vaccines, because the immune system's protection against certain germs wears off in time and needs to be renewed. These vaccines are called *booster shots.* One example of a booster shot is the tetanus shot.

There are two types of germs which vaccines protect against: bacteria and viruses. Some vaccines need to be given only once, and others have to be given several times to build up the body's defenses.

It is not possible to prevent all infections with vaccines. There is presently no vaccine, for example, to protect against the common cold or against chicken pox. There are many reasons for this. One is that certain infections, such as the common cold, are caused by a germ that exists in many slightly different forms. Each different form would require a different vaccine. Another reason is that it is not easy to develop vaccines that are both safe to use and effective in stimulating the child's immune system. Progress is being made all the time, however. Over the next five to ten years new vaccines for children will probably become widely available. A vaccine for chicken pox may be available soon.

Specific Vaccines

DPT: Stands for *diphtheria, pertussis, and tetanus vaccine.* Another name for pertussis is *whooping cough.*

TD: Contains tetanus vaccine and a smaller dose of diphtheria vaccine. This is the usual shot given for tetanus; a smaller dose of diphtheria is required for older children and adults. A tetanus shot should be given every 10 years to a fully immunized individual. It can be hazardous to receive tetanus shots too often.

MMR: Stands for *measles* (also called *red measles* or *10-day measles*), *mumps, and rubella vaccine.* Another name for rubella is *German measles.* This vaccine needs to be given only once.

OPV: Stands for *oral polio vaccine,* sometimes also abbreviated as TOPV. The *T* stands for *trivalent,* which indicates that there are three slightly different strains of the polio virus.

Hib: Stands for *Haemophilus influenza type b.* Hib is a germ which is the most common cause of life-threatening bacterial disease in young children. Hib-caused illnesses include: meningitis, pneumonia, and epiglottitis (see Chapter 2, "Breathing Problems". About one child in two hundred will be affected by a Hib disease before the age of 5.

  The Hib vaccine has been widely available only since mid-1985. If the Hib vaccine was not available when your child was 2 years old, he should receive the shot if he is under 6 years of age. The Hib vaccine is not necessary for children over the age of 6 years because it rarely affects individuals over this age.

  The Hib vaccine has also been termed the "H Flu" shot. Do not confuse H Flu with "the flu." *H Flu* is a bacteria, and *the flu* is caused by a type of virus. They are two completely different germs. The Hib or H Flu vaccine is *not* a flu shot.

One shot usually contains more than one vaccine. A DPT injection, for example, contains three different vaccines mixed together. A *TB skin test* (also called the *tine* test) is *not* a vaccine against tuberculosis (TB). It is a *test* to determine if someone has even been exposed to the tuberculosis germ.

Are Vaccines Safe?

This question concerns many parents. The issue boils down to whether a child is likely to suffer more harm from getting a vaccine than from not getting a vaccine.

No vaccine is completely safe. Many children experience side effects after being vaccinated. Usually these are relatively mild and do not cause permanent damage. Side effects are for the most part unavoidable because they are caused by the immune system's reaction to the vaccine.

DPT immunization may cause swelling and tenderness at the site of the injection. Fever and irritability can also occur. These symptoms usually last no longer than 2 days. The Hib vaccine will, in rare instances, cause swelling and tenderness at the site of the injection, or a mild fever. These symptoms usually last no longer than 1 or 2 days. The MMR vaccine occasionally causes mild fever and rash which begins 7 to 10 days after the immunization and lasts 2 or 3 days.

If your child has received an immunization and has developed side effects shortly thereafter, you should call your doctor or clinic if:

1. Any symptoms last longer than 48 hours.

2. Fever goes over 105° Fahrenheit (40.5° Celsius).

3. Persistent crying or irritability lasts more than 3 hours.

Should Your Child Receive DPT Shots?

There has recently been a great deal of controversy surrounding DPT shots. Almost all authorities agree that DPT shots *should* be given.

Concerns have been voiced regarding the P, or pertussis-containing component, of DPT shots. Pertussis, or whooping cough, can cause such severe fits of coughing that oxygen is prevented from getting to the brain. When this occurs, severe brain damage and even death are possible.

Brain damage can result from the pertussis vaccine as well. This is an extremely rare event, however, occurring only once in every 310,000 doses. A child who *does not* receive pertussis vaccine is *10 times more likely* to suffer severe brain damage or death than a child who is immunized.

Despite what you may have read or seen on television, there is no established scientific evidence that the pertussis vaccine causes sudden infant death syndrome (SIDS). In fact, the study from the National Institutes of Health indicates that SIDS is *8 times less likely* to occur in infants who have recently received DPT.

Much of the confusion regarding SIDS and DPT shots has occurred because the first year of life is the time when SIDS happens and it is also the time when the first three DPT shots are given. This does not mean that SIDS and DPT shots are related. An example may help demonstrate this point: Infants commonly start to teethe and get their first tooth around 6 months of age. If one monitored all the millions of American children who were immunized every year, one would find that a certain number of children would begin to teethe within minutes or hours of receiving a DPT shot. This would not mean, however, that the shot caused the teething to begin.

Finally, do not assume that because everyone else's children have been immunized, your child can safely avoid receiving DPT shots. DPT shots do not remove the pertussis germ from the community. Immunized children do carry the germ without getting sick themselves. Children immunized with DPT can still pick up the pertussis germ and be contagious to unimmunized children.

If you have any further concerns or questions regarding immunizations, you should discuss them with your doctor at your child's next checkup.

When Your Child Should Be Immunized

Schedule for Immunization of Healthy Infants and Children
(Abbreviations for vaccines are explained on page 241.)

Age	Vaccine	Comment
2 months	DPT OPV	
4 months	DPT OPV	
6 months	DPT OPV	This third administration of OPV is optional.
12 months	TB skin test*	This is repeated at various intervals.
15 months	MMR	
18 months	DPT OPV	
2 years	Hib	
4 to 6 years	DPT OPV	
14 to 16 years	Td	This should be repeated every 10 years.

* As explained on page 241, this is not actually a vaccine.

This schedule is the one recommended by the American Academy of Pediatrics. It is used by most pediatricians and family practitioners in the United States.

Most children will be able to receive all their shots on schedule. However, in certain situations shots should be delayed. For example, if a child has an infection with fever, such as pneumonia, at the time of a scheduled immunization, the shot should not be given. The common cold, as long as fever is absent, is *not* a reason to put off a scheduled immunization. Children with major medical problems require special consideration, and some may never receive immunizations. The decision to give immunizations has to be made depending on the details of each child's specific situation.

Remember, if your child has a scheduled immunization postponed because of an infection with fever, see that your child gets that shot very soon after he or she is better.

Up-to-date immunization is a school-entrance requirement in most states. The record of immunization is an important document. Most physicians will give you a "shot book" in which to record your child's immunizations. Remember to bring it with you at each well-baby checkup (see sample on page 246). At the end of the book is a sheet you may wish to tear out and use for recording shots.

Your Child's Immunization (Shot) Record

	Date	*Doctor's Signature*
DPT		
Td		
OPV		
MMR		
Hib		
TB skin test		

45. *Physical Fitness*

Over the past few decades the United States has become a sports- and fitness-oriented nation. Thus, it is surprising to learn that, according to a recent national study, American schoolchildren are *fatter and less fit today* than they were in the 1960s, and that only half of them get the exercise they need to stay healthy as adults.

What is the explanation for this paradox? How can we be more interested in sports, and have less active and healthy children? The primary reason seems to be that emphasis is being placed on competitive team sports rather than on physical fitness as such.

Football, basketball, baseball, and other competitive sports by themselves do not develop lifelong physical fitness in the school athlete. Kids need to learn skills and habits they can use by themselves that will allow them to stay physically fit for life. Activities such as running, swimming, skating, dancing, and aerobic exercise require a minimum of skill and expense and provide excellent exercise for lifelong fitness.

How Much Exercise?

At present the recommendation of cardiologists and sports physicians is for twenty minutes of vigorous physical activity three times per week. This is the minimum requirement to keep the heart, lungs, and circulatory system in good condition.

When and How to Start

The best time to start introducing regular exercise is around junior high school age. At this age children are beginning to participate less in school-based physical education, and they are old enough to start taking responsibility for their own health and fitness.

A good way to start is by making exercise a regular family activity so that everyone benefits. Also, it is much easier to exercise with others than alone; you are less conscious of the tedious and boring aspects of exercise.

The hardest part of exercise is to stick with it day in and day out. Exercise is only of benefit if it is done on a regular basis. It should become a lifelong habit for your children. They are most likely to exercise consistently if they see you doing so.

If you are over 35 years of age, you should first check with your doctor before starting an exercise program.

A Word about Smoking

Finally, and most important of all, if anyone in the family *smokes cigarettes*, get the person to *stop*.

Smoking causes lung cancer, emphysema, heart attacks, and other serious illnesses. Women who smoke during pregnancy are much more likely to have small, sickly infants. Smoking is by far the leading cause of preventable adult deaths in the United States.

IV. *Medical Terms*

This glossary is divided into the following categories:

- Types of doctors and other medical personnel
- Medical tests and procedures
- Diseases and illnesses
- Other medical terms

Many of the medical terms listed below are used in hospitals. Understanding certain terms will make the hospital experience less bewildering for you. At times doctors slip into medical language when talking to patients and parents. If you are ever unsure of what a doctor has told you, ask him or her to kindly repeat it in a nontechnical way.

The section on diseases discusses several illnesses which are not discussed elsewhere in the book. If you are looking up a disease and it is not mentioned in this section, check the index.

Types of Doctors and Other Medical Personnel

Attending physician: A doctor who has finished all of his or her training. The attending doctor may work for the hospital or be in private practice. This doctor is the most senior person involved in the care of patients and supervises the overall care of patients.

Cardiologist (pronounced: card ee *ahl* uh just): A doctor who specializes in the care of the heart.

Chief resident: The most senior house officer (*see* House officer). Each specialty usually has its own chief resident. For example, there might be a chief surgical resident and a chief pediatric resident.

Gastroenterologist (pronounced: *gas* tro ent er *rahl* uh just): A doctor who specializes in the care of the stomach, intestines, and other parts of the digestive system.

Hematologist (pronounced: he muh *tahl* uh just): A doctor who treats blood problems.

House officer: This is the term for a doctor in training who works for a hospital. Interns and residents are house officers.

Intern: A doctor who is in the first year of training: a type of house officer (*see* House officer).

Medical student: Someone in medical school studying to be a doctor. Senior medical students often are given a great deal of responsibility under the supervision of senior doctors.

Neonatologist (pronounced: knee uh nate *ahl* uh just): A pediatrician who specializes in the care of newborn and premature infants.

Nephrologist (pronounced: nih *frahl* uh just): A doctor who specializes in the care of the kidneys.

Neurologist (pronounced: nyuh *rahl* uh just): A doctor who specializes in the care of the brain, nerves, and muscles.

Obstetrician (pronounced: obb stuh *trish* un): A doctor who specializes in the care of pregnant women and the delivery of infants.

Oncologist (pronounced: on *kahl* uh just): A doctor who treats cancer.

Ophthalmologist (pronounced: ahf thal *mahl* uh just): A physician who specializes in the care of the eye. He or she can prescribe corrective glasses, treat and diagnose eye diseases, and perform eye surgery.

Optician (pronounced: opp *tish* un): A person who makes and sells eyeglasses. An optician can fill, but not write, a prescription for corrective glasses.

Optometrist (pronounced: opp *tom* uh trust): A person who can test the eyes for defects of vision in order to prescribe glasses.

Orthopedist (pronounced: or thuh *peed* ust): A doctor who specializes in the care of the bones.

Pediatrician (pronounced: *peed* ee uh *trish* un): A doctor who specializes in the care of infants, children, and adolescents (teenagers).

Physician: A person who is legally qualified to practice medicine; in other words, a doctor of medicine.

Psychiatrist (pronounced: suh *kye* uh trust): A doctor who specializes in treating stress and emotional problems.

Psychologist (pronounced: sigh *kahl* uh just): A person trained to work with people who have emotional problems or people who are under stress. A psychologist is not a physician.

Resident: A resident is a doctor in training who has finished the first year of training (internship); a type of house officer (*see* House officer).

Urologist (pronounced: yuh *rahl* uh just): A surgeon who specializes in the treatment of kidney, bladder, and urination problems.

Medical Tests and Procedures

Anesthesia (pronounced: an us *thee* zhuh): Means "the loss of feeling or sensation." The term *anesthesia* is most commonly used to describe the loss of pain sensation which is produced by medicines before surgery or other painful procedures.

Local anesthesia is produced by injecting a numbing medicine into the area which is to be worked upon, as for example, when a dentist injects a local anesthetic into the gums before filling a cavity. General anesthesia is given in the operating room just before surgery or other procedure; its purpose is to render the patient unconscious. Infants and young children may require general anesthesia for certain special tests because they cannot be expected to cooperate and hold still for a prolonged period.

Blood gas: A test that tells how well the lungs and heart are working. It gives the levels of oxygen and carbon dioxide as well as acid and base in the bloodstream. Blood for this test is usually taken from an artery in the arm; this can be very painful at times. A blood gas is a very safe test.

Blood tests or blood work: Refers to a group of tests that analyze different contents of the blood. Different tests give the level in the bloodstream of a medicine, mineral, or other substance such as an enzyme or sugar. Another test may look at cells in the bloodstream. Blood for these tests is taken by small needles which pierce through the skin and enter a vein, usually a vein in an arm. It may be necessary to use veins of the feet or scalp in small children and infants. A tourniquet is used to make the vein fatter and therefore easier to locate and pierce. These tests range from being slightly uncomfortable to moderately painful. They are very safe.

CBC: A blood test that analyzes the different types of cells in the blood. A CBC measures the levels of white blood cells, red blood cells, and platelets. White blood cells fight infection. Red blood cells carry oxygen. Too few red blood cells causes anemia. Platelets help stop bleeding.

CT scan or CAT scan: A computerized x-ray, often used to show the soft tissues inside the body, something a plain x-ray does poorly. A sedative medicine is often given to infants and young children before a CT scan, because the patient must lie very still during the scan.

Sometimes a special dye called *contrast* is used to improve the detail of CT scans. A temporary injection into a vein is needed when using contrast; this can be painful at times. Very rarely, a child will have an allergic reaction to the contrast dye. The dye cannot be given to certain children who have severe kidney problems.

CT scanning is an extremely safe procedure. The scanning itself is completely painless.

Cystoscopy (pronounced: sis tuh *skahp* ee): A test in which a doctor places a small, flexible plastic tube through the urethra (the opening where urine leaves the body), and into the bladder. The doctor then looks into the bladder to see if there is any problem. Children usually have general anesthesia for this test. Cystoscopy is safe and rarely painful.

Echocardiogram: A way of using sound waves to look at the heart. Certain types of echocardiograms can actually show the heart beating. This test is safe and painless.

EEG: Stands for *electroencephalogram*, sometimes referred to as a *brain wave test*, which measures the electric activity of the brain. Small pieces of metal, called *electrodes*, are taped or temporarily glued to the scalp. Infants and young children are often given medicine to make them sleepy before an EEG. This test is most often used to diagnose seizures. It is safe and painless.

EKG: Stands for *electrocardiogram*, which measures the electric activity of the heart. Small, flat pieces of metal, called *electrodes*, are placed on several parts of the body. This is a safe and painless test.

Enema: A technique for introducing fluid into the intestines. A small rubber or plastic tube is passed through the anus (the opening through which bowel movements pass), into the lowest part of the intestines; the tube is connected to a fluid container. The fluid is either squirted or dripped in through the anus. This can be done as a treatment, for example, to cleanse the bowels in severe cases of constipation, or before surgery. An enema can also be used as a diagnostic test. A *barium enema* is an x-ray test to visualize the lower intestines. Barium is a material that shows up well on x-rays. Enemas are uncomfortable and unpleasant but rarely painful. They are very safe when performed properly.

MRI: A new technique for obtaining extremely detailed pictures of the inside of the body. MRI utilizes fast-moving magnetic fields to create images. It can take a while for the pictures to be assembled. MRI is a safe and painless procedure. Children may require medicines to make them sleepy before the test.

Sonogram: *See* Ultrasound.

Spinal tap: A procedure in which a small needle is inserted into the back, between the bones of the spine, into the space containing spinal fluid. A small amount of spinal fluid, equivalent to 1 or 2 teaspoons, is then removed. Spinal fluid is the fluid which bathes the brain and spinal cord. The fluid is tested for evidence of infection and other abnormalities.

Spinal taps are generally safe procedures; they do not cause a child to become paralyzed. In rare conditions where there is increased pressure on the brain, as in brain tumors, a spinal tap can be dangerous. A child will have clear signs of increased pressure which your doctor can spot easily.

A spinal tap is necessary when meningitis is suspected. It is the *only* way to tell if someone has meningitis. Spinal taps can be uncomfortable and at times painful. However, when a life-threatening meningitis infection is suspected, there is no reason to delay performing a spinal tap.

The medical term for spinal tap is *lumbar puncture*. Spinal fluid is also called *CSF*, which stands for *cerebrospinal* (pronounced: suh ree bro *spine* ul) fluid.

Transfusion: A procedure for giving a patient blood or blood products through a vein.

Ultrasound: A way of using sound waves to look inside the body. It is particularly useful for pregnant women because it is considered to be safer than x-rays. It may be mildly uncomfortable, but it is not painful. This is a safe test, and to date there is no evidence that ultrasound harms the fetus. Ultrasound may also be used to study the brain of a newborn infant. In this situation, the ultrasound pictures are taken through the soft spot on the head. *Sonogram* is another term for ultrasound.

X-ray: A way of taking pictures of structures inside the body. It uses extremely small amounts of radiation and a special type of film. When it is necessary to take an x-ray, the risk of radiation is much less harmful to your child than the disease or injury he or she may have. X-rays can be harmful to a fetus, however, so pregnant women should have x-rays only in emergency situations. X-rays have many important uses. They are particularly good at showing broken bones. X-rays are not painful unless they require moving injured body parts.

Diseases and Illnesses

This section discusses illnesses that are not dealt with elsewhere in the book. If you are looking for information about a disease or illness and it is not mentioned below, check the index.

Anemia (pronounced: uh *knee* me uh): The condition where blood is too thin. Blood is made up of blood cells and fluid. The fluid is called *plasma*. If blood does not contain enough red blood cels, anemia results. There are many different causes of anemia. The most common cause of anemia in childhood is a deficiency of iron.

Cerebral palsy: A condition of poor motor development. Cerebral palsy has a wide range of severity, from a moderate degree of clumsiness to total paralysis. Cerebral palsy does not get worse over time.

Cystic fibrosis: A rare disease characterized by poor weight gain in infancy; frequent lung infections; and frequent, greasy bowel movements.

Diabetes: A disease in which the body is unable to handle sugar properly. Diabetes usually starts with weight loss, unusual thirst and frequent drinking of liquids, unusually frequent urination, abdominal pains, and leg cramps. Insulin is given to diabetic children to allow them to metabolize sugar properly.

Children with diabetes can learn at home to test their urine and blood (from a pinprick of the finger) for sugar levels. Insulin dosages may have to be adjusted depending on the levels of sugar in the urine and blood. Many diabetic children can give themselves their own insulin injections. Insulin cannot be given by mouth. Children with diabetes must also follow special diets.

Teamwork by the diabetic child, parents, doctors, dieticians, nurses, and nurse clinicians is required for children to be able to keep the level of sugar in the blood at a proper level. Most children with diabetes lead active, productive, happy lives.

Hypertension: High blood pressure. It does not mean "severe anxiety" or "a worried state."

Sepsis (pronounced: *sep* suss): The condition where an overwhelming infection has occurred and large numbers of germs have spread throughout the bloodstream.

Shock: A condition of severely low blood pressure. Shock can occur as a result of massive bleeding, severe dehydration, overwhelming infection, or heart failure. The medical term *shock* does not mean "fainting spell," "severe fright," or "a state of being startled."

URI: Stands for *upper respiratory infection.* A URI is a cold.

UTI: Stands for *urinary tract infection.* This refers to an infection of the bladder or the tubes connecting the bladder to the kidneys.

Other Medical Terms

Acetaminophen (pronounced: uh *seat* uh *min* uh fun): The generic term for a nonaspirin pain-reliever and fever medicine.

Acute: Beginning suddenly or quickly over minutes to days (*compare with* Chronic).

Antibiotic: A medicine that kills bacteria. Penicillin is one type of antibiotic. Antibiotics are *useless* against viruses. Viruses, another type of germ, cause such illnesses as the common cold and chicken pox.

Anus: The opening of the intestines through which bowel movements pass.

Bilateral: A term meaning "both" or "both sides." For example, *bilateral ear infection* means "an infection in both ears."

Cardiac: A term meaning "of the heart." For example, *cardiac disease* means "heart disease."

Catheter (pronounced: *kath* ut ur): A tube used in medical procedures, usually made of plastic or rubber.

Chronic: A term meaning "beginning slowly" or "lasting a long time" (*compare with* Acute).

Diagnosis: The identification of the disease a person has.

Fistula (pronounced: *fiss* chuh luh): An abnormal opening or passage. A bullet creates a fistula when it passes through the body.

GI: Stands for *gastrointestinal,* meaning "something pertaining to the digestive system."

Hemorrhage: A condition of bleeding.

Hepatic (pronounced: hih *pat* ik): A term meaning "of the liver." For example, *hepatic failure* means "liver failure."

Hernia: Any abnormal bulge in tissue.

IM: Stands for *intramuscular,* meaning "in the muscle." A medicine given as a shot is given IM.

Infarct and infarction (pronounced: *in* farkt; in *fark* shun): A localized area of tissue which is dead or dying because it has been deprived of its blood supply.

Inflammation: A condition marked by pain, redness, tenderness, swelling, and heat. Inflammation usually occurs as the body's reaction to an injury or infection.

Intubation (pronounced: in tyoo *bay* shun): Insertion of a breathing tube into the mouth, through the voice box, and down into the windpipe. Intubation must be performed before a respirator can be used.

IV: Stands for *intravenous,* meaning "in the vein." Medicines and fluids are often given IV. The term *IV* is also used to refer to the needle and tubing used to give medicines or fluids intravenously. Fluids are often given IV to treat dehydration and to feed children who cannot take anything by mouth for a few days.

IVs are usually placed into veins of the hands or forearms. Infants and small children will often require an IV in the scalp or feet. It can take great skill to put an IV into an infant. A needle or small plastic catheter is threaded into a vein after the skin is pierced. The catheter or needle piercing the skin has to be firmly stabilized and protected. When IVs "blow," meaning that the vein has begun to leak, the area around the needle or catheter becomes very puffy. The puffiness is not permanent. A blown IV has to be changed.

It can be quite painful to have an IV placed and many attempts may be necessary with infants and younger children. Once in place, an IV is uncomfortable but usually not painful. Children will try to pull their IVs out. It is important that careful attention be paid to keeping the IV site protected.

Lymph nodes: Lymph nodes are part of the body's defense system. When they become large and painful, they are actively fighting infection. Lymph nodes are located throughout the body. They can be felt in the neck and groin, for example. We say that a child has swollen "glands," but these are actually lymph nodes in the neck which have enlarged due to a cold or sore throat.

Negative: A negative test result means that nothing abnormal was detected. Thus, it is usually a good result. For example, the statement, "The spinal tap was completely negative," indicates that the results of the spinal tap showed everything to be completely normal (*compared with* Positive).

Neonate (pronounced: *knee* uh nate): An infant under 1 month of age.

NPO: Shorthand for saying, "Patient is to get nothing by mouth."

Plasma: The fluid part of blood, which does not contain any cells.

Platelets (pronounced: *plate* luts): Small blood cells which help blood to clot.

PO: Means "by mouth," or "orally." Many medicines can be given PO.

Positive: A positive test result means that something abnormal was detected. For example, the statement, "The chest x-ray was positive for pneumonia," indicates that there was evidence of pneumonia on the chest x-ray (*compare with* Negative).

PRN: Means "as needed." For example, a doctor may order "Acetaminophen every 4 hours PRN pain."

Prognosis: A forecast of the course of a disease.

Pulmonary (pronounced: *pull* muh nehr ee): A term meaning "of the lungs." For example, *pulmonary disease* means "lung disease."

RBC: Stands for *red blood cell*. Red blood cells carry oxygen from the lungs to the body tissues.

Rectum: The last part of the intestines just before the anus.

Renal: Term meaning "of the kidneys." For example, *renal transplant* means "kidney transplant."

Respirator and ventilator: Terms referring to breathing machines. These machines help the lungs work.

Sedative: Any medicine which makes a patient sleepy.

Ulcer: A sore that creates an open depression or erosion in the skin or a body cavity. It most commonly refers to a sore inside the stomach or the upper intestines.

Ureter (pronounced: *yuhr* ut ur): A tube of the body that takes urine from the kidney into the bladder. There are normally two ureters, one from each kidney.

Urethra (pronounced: yuh *ree* thruh): The tube that carries urine from the bladder out of the body.

W.B.C.: Stands for *white blood cell*. These cells are part of the body's defense against infection.

References

Sources used in preparation of this book include:

Kempke CH, Silver HK, O'Brien D (eds): *Current Pediatric Diagnosis & Treatment*, 8th ed. Los Altos, Lange, 1984.

Vaughan VC, McKay RJ, Behrman RE, Nelson WE (eds): *Nelson Textbook of Pediatrics*, 12th ed. Philadelphia, Saunders, 1983.

Rudolph AM, Hoffman JIE, Axelrod S (eds): *Pediatrics*, 17th ed. Norwalk, Appleton-Century Crofts, 1982.

National Safety Council: Our Child's World.

American Academy of Pediatrics: Red Book.

American Academy of Pediatrics: TIPP: The injury prevention program.

American Academy of Pediatrics: Pediatric Patient Education: Challenge for the 80's. *Pediatrics* 1984; 74(Suppl.).

Index

Splints and Slings (repeat from p. 14)

(repeat from p. 14)

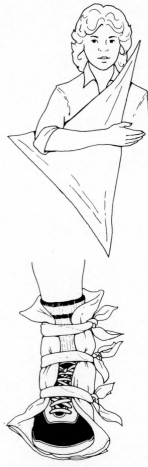

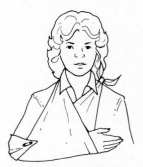

How to make a sling for shoulder, collarbone, or arm injuries.

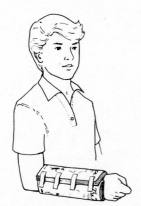

Arm splint using a newspaper or magazine and tape.

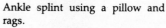

Ankle splint using a pillow and rags.

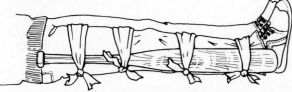

Leg splint using a baseball bat and rags.

(cut on this line)

(cut on this line)

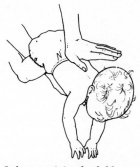

Infant receiving back blows.

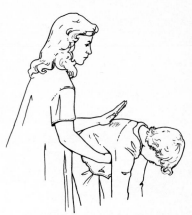

Child receiving back blows.

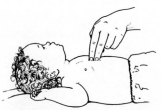

Infant receiving chest compressions. (*Note:* Only two fingers are used.)

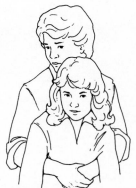

Child receiving abdominal thrusts. (*Note:* Direction of thrust is an inward and upward motion.)

(*Repeat from p. 29*)

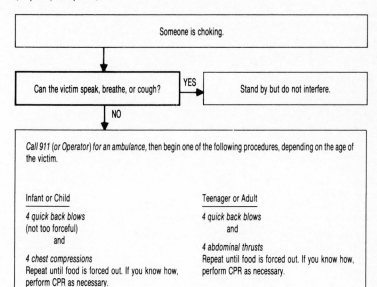

Someone is choking.

Can the victim speak, breathe, or cough? → **YES** → Stand by but do not interfere.

NO

Call 911 (or Operator) for an ambulance, then begin one of the following procedures, depending on the age of the victim.

Infant or Child

4 quick back blows
(not too forceful)
    and

4 chest compressions
Repeat until food is forced out. If you know how, perform CPR as necessary.

Teenager or Adult

4 quick back blows
    and

4 abdominal thrusts
Repeat until food is forced out. If you know how, perform CPR as necessary.

Clear the food or object from the child's mouth *only* if clearly visible and accessible. *Be careful* not to inadvertently push the object further into the child's throat.

(*Repeat from p. 246*)

Your Child's Immunization (Shot) Record

	Date	Doctor's Signature
DPT	_____	_____
	_____	_____
	_____	_____
	_____	_____
	_____	_____
Td	_____	_____
OPV	_____	_____
	_____	_____
	_____	_____
	_____	_____
	_____	_____
MMR	_____	_____
Hib	_____	_____
TB skin test	_____	_____
	_____	_____
	_____	_____
	_____	_____

(cut on this line)